D0150679

DR. KELLON'S
GUIDE
TO
FIRST AID
FOR
HORSES

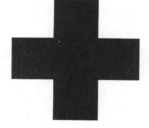

by

ELEANOR KELLON, VMD

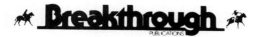

PUBLICATIONS

Special thanks to Dr. Corinne Sweeney,
Dr. Jill Beech and Dr. James Orsini
of the New Bolton Center
for contributing color photographs.

For information address:

Breakthrough Publications, Inc.
www.booksonhorses.com

International Standard Book Number: 0-914327-29-1

Designed by Jacques Chazaud
Illustrations by Kip Carter
Original black and white photos by Tricia Booker

Reprinted in 2004 by Imprelibros S.A.

The following products mentioned in this book are
Registered in the U.S. Patent and Trademark
Office:

Acepromazine, Alka Seltzer, A-H solution, Atro-
pine, Banamine, Betadine, Blukote, Fleet's Enema,
Dipyrone, Dyrex, Hexachloraphene, Ivermectin,
Jenotone, K-Y Jelly, PHisoHex, PHisoDerm, Phe-
nothiazine, Phenylbutazone, Procaine, Promazine,
Q-Tips, Rompun, Scarlet-Red, Telfa, Tetracycline,
Topazone, Torbutrol, Tribrissin, Vetwrap, Vicks,
Xylazine

A Message From the Author and the Publisher

This book is not intended to be used as a substitute for veterinary care, or as a "do-it-yourself" manual. The situations covered are genuine emergencies (with the exception of some entries that the owner or other caretaker might confuse for an emergency) and therefore warrant a visit by the veterinarian. In some instances, guidelines have been given on how long it would be acceptable to wait before having the veterinarian call. However, this is based strictly on average, uncomplicated cases and should not be used as a hard and fast rule.

The veterinarian should be contacted as soon as possible if any of the problems described herein are encountered. It is always preferable to clear any recommended procedures or medications with the veterinarian prior to implementing them. Individual animals or special circumstances might dictate special precautions or other measures.

It is recommended that this book be reviewed prior to encountering any emergency. Any unfamiliar techniques, procedures or medications should be discussed with your veterinarian to avoid problems should that emergency occur. If you are unsure about the diagnosis of the problem, the techniques or procedures recommended or any medication (or its administration), WAIT FOR THE VETERINARIAN.

The success of medical treatments depends upon many factors, including, but not limited to, proper diagnosis, familiarity with any idiosyncracies of the individual animal, proficiency of the person providing the treatment and drug actions/reactions/interactions, which are not under the control of the author or the publisher of this guide. Neither Breakthrough Publications nor Dr. Eleanor Kellon shall be liable to any person for damage resulting from reliance on any information contained in DR. KELLON'S GUIDE TO FIRST AID FOR HORSES whether with respect to diagnosis, drug dosages, treatment procedures, or by reason of any misstatement or inadvertent error contained herein.

Contents

CHAPTER I

Guidelines

The purpose of this book is to provide a quick and easy reference to conditions that require emergency treatment, and to advise what you can do until the veterinarian arrives. It is not intended to replace diagnosis and treatment by your veterinarian. However, it will offer guidelines to be followed in determining what the horse's problem could be and suggest information which should be given to the veterinarian as soon as you call. There are easy-to-follow instructions on what emergency treatments you can perform.

The appendices also contain a list of the general signs of serious illness as well as illustrations on how to perform various routine procedures, such as restraint, injections, administration of eye medications, and application of bandages. These will be helpful both in the emergency situation and when carrying out the follow up treatment recommended by your veterinarian.

DR. KELLON'S GUIDE TO FIRST AID FOR HORSES

CHAPTER II

Being Prepared

Everyone wonders how he or she might handle an emergency situation, whether he or she would panic or rush right in and be heroic. In fact, those who perform best under emergency situations are usually the people who know what to do. Advance preparation, good organization and a cool head are all needed.

It is recommended that you become very familiar with this book before you actually need it. This will make it easier for you to find the information you need quickly and may prevent your making a mistake if the book is not at hand the moment you need it. (For example, you might remember that it is dangerous to force a horse that is tied up to walk.) Advance preparation should also include assembling your first aid supplies and filling in emergency phone numbers.

There are many things you, as the owner or caretaker, can do before the veterinarian arrives. In addition to providing emergency treatments, you can make the veterinarian's job easier by assembling vital pieces of information necessary to make a diagnosis. The Emergency Information Sheet (Appendix 1) lists the things the veterinarian will want to know. It is most helpful if you have most of this data on hand when you call the veterinarian, although in certain situations, as when a horse is experiencing heavy arterial bleeding, basic information (such as "My horse is bleeding from an artery in his leg, is lying flat on the ground and trembling") will have to do.

The techniques for taking pulse and temperature are illustrated in Appendix 7. A respiratory rate is obtained simply by counting how many times the horse's chest moves in and out over a minute.

The color of the mucous membranes (such as the gums) also provides important clues to the horse's overall condition, with a very pale or white color indicating blood loss; a bright red color indicating a toxic condition; a grey-blue color indicating severe shock; and a bright

Checking the mucous membranes of the mouth for color.

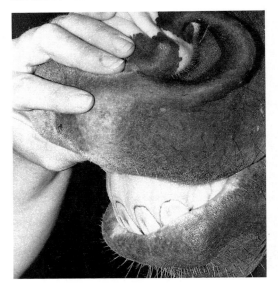

yellow color, possibly indicating liver disease. Also, applying light pressure to the mucous membranes can reveal clues to the horse's health. Light pressure causes the mucous membranes to blanch. The amount of time it takes the color to return (usually around one to two seconds) is called the capillary refill time. In shock-like states, the capillary refill time is prolonged. (You can practice this technique on your own finger or toe nails. The pressure needed to result in a white spot is the same pressure to apply to a horse's gums.)

Make note of anything else abnormal about the horse's behavior and appearance. This information may be specific, such as refusal to open an eye and tearing, or, more general, such as depression, trembling, or sweating. Everything you note could be important, so be observant. Check the feed bin, water bucket and hay supply. Observe the stall for character and quantity of urine and feces. Observe the bedding for any signs of thrashing or struggling around. If you know when the horse first became ill or injured, record this. If not, state when he was last seen well and when he was found ill.

After the veterinarian has been called, continue with the emergency treatments recommended and/or those ordered by your veterinarian. While waiting for the veterinarian to arrive, you should also record the TPR (temperature, pulse and respiration) at 15- to 20-minute intervals in life-threatening situations, check the mucous membranes, and note any change in symptoms. Use your permanent barn records or keep a clipboard with a pad of paper and pen with your other first aid supplies.

Finally, when you have a minute, try to think of anything that might have caused or contributed to the problem, or of any similar episodes in the past, and write them down so you don't forget to mention them in the commotion after the veterinarian arrives. Never rely on your memory during an emergency. There is simply too much going on to remember all these pieces of information.

As for keeping a cool head, nothing will calm you down quicker than having something to do and getting on with it. Company helps too, so telephone for nearby help as soon as you reach the veterinarian. Do not hesitate to enlist the help of paramedics, the fire department, or similar services if the animal is trapped. They may not be familiar with horses, but they will know how best to free a trapped horse and can assist you with basic first aid techniques.

NORMAL VALUES—TPR (TEMPERATURE, PULSE AND RESPIRATION)

Temperature: 98° to 100°

Pulse: 44 (Range high 20's to low 40's)

Respiration: 8 to 16

All values are given for animals at rest. Foals will tend to run in the upper ranges. Weather conditions will also affect values (i.e. higher on hot days). Excitement and fear will quickly elevate pulse and respiration, which will just as quickly return to normal as the animal is quieted.

CHAPTER III

How to Use This Book

This book is organized by chapters on specific types of problems (e.g. Wounds, Bleeding, Burns, etc.) or on specific anatomical areas (e.g. Eyes) and organ systems (e.g. Disorders of Eating and Colic). At the beginning of each chapter is an alphabetical list of symptoms that allows you to turn immediately to those sections of the chapter which might pertain to your horse's problems. For example, "cough" in the chapter on Breathing Problems will refer you to page 98. If your horse also has "nasal discharge," this keys you to page 99.

If you are unsure about what organ system your horse's symptoms are related to, turn to the complete index at the end of the book. This will also refer you to any other organ system that you may not have realized may be involved in the problem. For example, "salivation" ("drooling," "foaming at the mouth") will refer you to the chapter on Disorders of Eating, as well as to the chapters on Collapse/ Seizures and Disorders of Balance. (botulism and rabies).

The text of each chapter is organized to show a list of conditions on the left-hand side of the page and the possible causes, with emergency treatments, on the right-hand side. The page numbers of pertinent illustrations will be given under symptoms and/or treatment, when appropriate.

The sections are also keyed by a system of stars as follows:

.   serious illness, get attention within 24 hours;

..   requires veterinary attention that day;

...   potentially life-threatening, seek immediate veterinary attention.

CHAPTER IV

Restraint of the Ill or Injured Horse

Before initiating any emergency treatments, or even examining the horse, it is necessary to assess his state of mind and establish adequate restraint. Horses vary in their response to pain and frightening circumstances. For example, a trapped horse, whether entangled in barbed wire, trapped in a trailer accident or simply cast in his stall, may be struggling wildly—or the horse may be lying perfectly still, almost in a trance.

A horse that is frantic may be dangerous to himself and to anyone who attempts to approach him. Before approaching the animal, be certain you have his attention. Keeping a safe distance, locate yourself close to his head (not his tail) and speak to him softly. Continue to make attempts to get the horse's attention by speaking softly. This will often calm the horse enough for you to approach. If the horse will not quiet down and seems totally unaware of your presence, do not attempt to go closer until you have help. The horse that seems calm, perhaps even too calm under the circumstances, may very well be in a state of shock, or afraid that any move he makes will cause pain. Such a horse must also be handled very carefully, as he may explode at any moment.

For example, I recall a carriage horse that was tied to a hitching post and out of sight. Suddenly a loud crash was heard and the horse was found lying flat on the ground and not moving. Her breathing was very slow and regular, pulse normal. The only thing moving was her eyes. Help was assembled and the harness loosened. As the carriage was being pulled back the horse suddenly began lurching violently and threw herself forward, only to collapse again. It was immediately obvious that she had somehow managed to impale herself on one of the shafts, which had been driven into her underarm and along the chest wall for a distance of approximately eight inches. This horse knew, as many do, that struggling under the circumstances could easily have injured her further. However, the minute she was released (and/or when she felt the pain of the shaft being removed), the instinct to flee was overwhelming.

This same mare is a good example of how a horse in shock should be handled. After the initial release, the mare was trembling badly and very shaky on her feet. Her gums were extremely white and she was indifferent to the people and things around her, also refusing to eat or drink. There was initial concern she might be bleeding internally, but her strong and steady normal pulse argued against this. The horse was in a state of shock. triggered by her severe injury. During this time, it was possible to carefully examine, probe, clean and flush her wound with no restraint other than a lead shank. She even showed virtually no reaction to the injection of local anesthesia prior to suturing the wound. However, after general supportive measures of blanketing the mare and administering a large dose of phenylbutazone to ease her pain, the situation became quite different and she violently resisted any attempt to even approach the area of the injury. She was a very large mare and quite used to having her own way, so it was necessary to use a twitch for the next three days of treatments. After that time, the pain had eased enough that treatments could again be managed with only a lead shank.

To summarize, proper assessment of the horse's state of mind, while unpredictable, is essential to achieving control. The horse must not be approached until you have his attention. Once you have made contact, restraint should be appropriate to the degree of resistance the horse is showing. The depressed, "shocky" horse does not need to be twitched in most cases. In fact, to do so is itself an unnecessary stress to the already over-stressed animal. On the other hand, the horse that actively resists your treatment will need effective restraint for his own good and the safety of all.

Methods of Restraint

The simplest method of restraint is the lead shank, simply clipped to the bottom of the halter. Basically, this keeps the horse from moving around and allows the handler to manipulate him in any direction desired. The handler should stand just in front of the shoulder, never directly in front of the horse (he could strike) and on the same side as the veterinarian or other person treating or examining the horse. This makes it possible to pull the horse's body away from the person working on him, should the horse act up.

A variation of the simple shank is a chain lead shank, with the chain run over or under the nose. This works well for horses that fidget around or are likely to try their luck at avoiding treatment but do not really require a twitch. When held quietly, the chain does not bother the horse. However, should more restraint be needed, a few quick jerks will get the horse's attention. One drawback here is that activating the effect of the chain tends to make the horse back up or even rear.

Chains can also be used in the mouth (passed through the mouth like a bit and hooked to the halter ring on the opposite side). Most horses will respect this almost as much as a twitch. It is very effective without actually injuring the horse in any way. It is most effectively used when the handler gives a few small jerks to get the horse's attention prior to the start of treatments and then keeps a little tension on the shank until the horse is resigned to being treated.

A more severe use of the chain shank, usually reserved for horses that cannot be twitched and for some reason should not be tranquilized, is running a chain on the gum, under the upper lip. Chains placed on the sensitive gums can cause significant pain and even bleeding if the horse fights it (as many will do). However, once the initial fight is over, the degree of restraint is equivalent to twitching, provided a slight tension is kept on the chain (if allowed to go slack it may slip off and into the mouth).

The use of chains for restraint should only be done by people experienced with this tech-

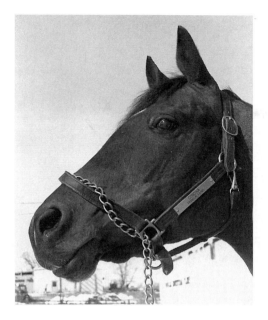

Uses of chain shank in restraint.

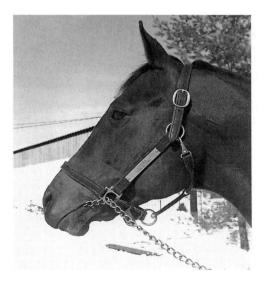

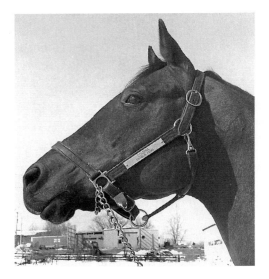

nique. When used too vigorously, or not convincingly enough, the horse is likely to fight.

The twitch is a very effective device for achieving control. Several types are available, including short and long-handled twitches with rope or chain on the end, and smooth metal twitches that are self-retaining and attach to the halter. The advantage of hand-held twitches is that they can be tightened or loosened as needed during the treatment. However, even the less severe self-retaining twitches work well under most circumstances and can be squeezed tighter by hand if need be.

Two people are needed to apply a twitch: one to hold the horse and the other to use the twitch. If you are right-handed, use your left hand to steady the horse's head by grasping the halter. Pass the loop of a hand-held twitch or the top portion of a self-retaining twitch over your right arm and grasp a generous portion of the horses upper lip/nose with your right hand. The left hand then releases the halter and passes the upper end of the twitch over the nose. The other handler should then begin to tighten or squeeze the twitch as the hand holding the nose is released to assume control of the twitch. The person controlling the twitch should then also take over the lead shank and position himself on the same side as the person doing treatments, as with a simple shank restraint. (See Appendix 8.)

When using a twitch, the most resistance is usually encountered during the procedure of trying to apply it. Once in place, the horse may attempt to back up or rear/toss his head to get free. However, after the initial resistance, most horses will stand quietly for routine treatments when twitched. The effectiveness of this device seems to transcend the actual discomfort it can cause. Some horses appear to actually doze off while twitched. In any event, do not hesitate to use this effective method to facilitate treatments.

Another method of restraint sometimes used very effectively is picking up a horse's leg. This is usually done when a horse has a limb problem and keeps lifting his leg, kicking, etc. when being worked on. When working on the hind end, pick up the front leg on the same side as the one being treated. When working on the forequarters, pick up the opposite front leg. One drawback of this maneuver is the very real possibility that the horse will continue to struggle and, being off balance, may actually fall. It is not recommended for high-strung horses and is most useful for those that simply tend to fidget around or lift a leg automatically every time it is touched.

Finally, there are tranquilizers—chemical restraint. Tranquilizers do not replace physical restraint, nor do they eliminate the possibility the horse will resist treatment. However, they do slow down the horse's responses and make him less likely to react to minor irritations. Pain will still generate a response, and even the tranquilized horse is quite capable of inflicting serious injury. Tranquilizers should only be administered by, or on the direction of, a veterinarian. For most non-veterinarians, the intramuscular route is preferable to the intravenous route, since accidental injection of some tranquilizers into an artery rather than a vein can cause severe reactions. This is a very real possibility with injections made high in the neck, where the needle may be injected at the wrong angle and penetrate an artery. With intramuscular injections, allow 15 to 20 minutes for the tranquilizer to take effect. See Appendix 4 for signs of adequate tranquilization.

Tranquilizers should never be used in horses that have sustained a significant blood loss, horses that appear to be in shock, horses that may have extensive internal injuries, or horses that may have a disturbed fluid balance (such as with colic, heat stroke, or urinary tract problems).

When properly used, tranquilizers are often the best approach to handling a fractious horse. By alleviating anxiety, they make the entire treatment process safer for both horse and handlers. It is often found that use of tranquilizers can be discontinued once the horse learns the routine of the treatment and what to expect and/or when the condition being treated is not as painful as in the acute stages.

SYMPTOM LIST

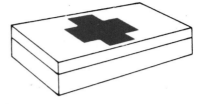

FIRST AID KIT

Iodine-based surgical scrub (soap)
  or
Hexachlorophene soap
Antibiotic ointment
Betadine ointment
Sterile gauze pads
Wound spray
Scarlet Red
Blukote
Topazone
Tetanus toxoid
Tetanus antitoxin
Quilted cotton leg bandages
Cloth or elasticized leg wraps
Antibiotics
  Injectable
    (Penicillin or penicillin combinations—no steroid)
  Oral
    (Tribrissen paste or pills)
Phenylbutazone (paste, pills or injectable)
Blanket
Epsom salts

CHAPTER V

Wounds

SUPERFICIAL WOUNDS (ABRASIONS AND LACERATIONS) *

Definition: Superficial wounds include abrasions and lacerations. Abrasions are brush-burn type injuries with loss of hair and minimal loss of skin, usually accompanied by oozing of clear fluids (serum) and some slow ooze of blood. Lacerations are injuries that penetrate the skin. With superficial lacerations, only the upper layers of skin are damaged. Typically, the edges of the wound will remain close together. There may be more bleeding than with abrasions but this is easily controlled by pressure, or it stops on its own within minutes.

Treatment: Hose the area with cool water for ten minutes. Follow this by gentle cleaning, using gauze and Betadine surgical scrub or a hexachlorophene soap (e.g. pHisoHex or pHisoDerm). If these are not available, use any gentle soap. Begin cleaning at the top of the wound and work down. (The horse may need restraint in addition to a lead shank or cross-ties.) Rinse well and inspect for any remaining debris or dirt. Allow area to dry and apply antibiotic ointment or Betadine ointment to wound. Apply a sterile gauze or Telfa pad over the wound and secure in place with either a partial bandage of the self-adhering type (e.g. Vetwrap) or a standard standing leg bandage. Injuries located on areas that cannot be bandaged should be dressed with the antibiotic ointment as above and repeatedly checked for any accumulating dirt, straw, etc., then recleaned and ointment reapplied as necessary. Do not use cotton balls or cotton when cleaning wounds, as the lint fibers may cause contamination. As an alternative treatment, Scarlet Red, Blukote, Topazone or any similar wound spray may be used and are less likely to attract dirt, as they form a dry surface. Do not use this type of medication (dry surface) if the wound looks as if it may need to be sutured.

Call the veterinarian if you have any question about whether the area might require sutures, or if swelling, heat and pain do not improve or worsen after 24 hours, or if a pus-like discharge develops, or if edges of a laceration are constantly being pulled apart

Severe abrasion with skin loss .

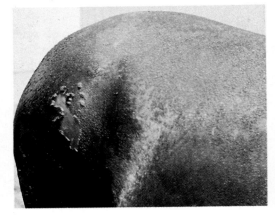

secondary to location of the injury (e.g. over the point of the hock).

Ideally, suturing needs to be done in the first six hours after the injury occurs. Longer intervals allow bacteria sufficient time to gain entry to the deep layers of tissue.

DEEP LACERATIONS **

Definition: Deep lacerations penetrate all layers of the skin and are characterized by the edges of the skin gaping apart. There may also be penetration of the injury to the level of the muscle or fascia (covering of muscle), tendons or even bone.

Treatment: (If bleeding, see chapter on Bleeding.)

Laceration through skin only:

Cleanse the area as described above for superficial wounds. Do not direct forceful streams of water directly at the wound as this may cause any dirt to become embedded. Large contaminating objects may be removed safely (e.g. twigs or leaves on the surface) but do not attempt to remove any embedded material— leave this to the veterinarian. When cleaning the wound with gauze, keep to the surface areas but allow the soap to run along the deeper layers. Rinse well, directing the water above the level of the wound and allowing it to run over the surface gently. Do not apply any spray or wound ointment (unless in water base) to the open wound. Moisten a sterile gauze dressing(s) with sterile saline solution, if available, and bandage as described above. If you do not have sterile bandaging materials, clean gauze or linen may be used. Do not use cotton or other high-lint materials, as fibers may contaminate the wound. If no lint-free bandaging material is available, it is best to leave the wound uncovered if the veterinarian is expected shortly, or to leave the horse in the wash stall or barn aisle until suitable covering can be obtained.

With deep wounds, very dirty wounds or wounds that are obviously not fresh when first discovered, it is often advisable to give an anti-biotic injection immediately. The old standby, for good reason, is procaine penicillin, or com-binations of penicillin and streptomycin. These are given intramuscularly. For those un-comfortable with the idea of giving injections, an excellent alternative is Tribrissen 400 Oral Paste, administered in the same way as paste formula worming drugs. Before giving any anti-biotic, get your veterinarian's approval. Keep the horse quiet and avoid any unnecessary moving around that could cause bleeding.

Check on the status of the horse's tetanus immunizations. If he has been vaccinated within the past year, a booster of tetanus tox-oid is advisable. If vaccination status is un-known, or last vaccination was over a year prior to injury, the horse will need both teta-nus toxoid and tetanus antitoxin protection. (Antitoxin begins to work immediately). These may be given at the same time but not at the same injection site.

If the horse is trembling, pale, and seems very depressed, blanket him and consult the veterinarian about administering pain medica-tion, such as phenylbutazone paste.

Laceration involving skin and muscle:

If the injury penetrates through to the muscular layer, moderate to heavy bleeding is often present and must be controlled first (see chapter on Bleeding.) If it is possible to wash the wound without causing bleeding to resume at an uncontrolled rate, proceed with cleansing as outlined above. When wounds involve avulsion of muscle — i.e. muscle torn away from its attachments and hanging loose — cleanse gently as best you can. Then attempt to manipulate the muscle back into the wound cavity, using a moist sponge, and proceed with bandaging. If bandaging is not possible, as with wounds on the chest or high on the hindquarters, stay with the horse to prevent his lying down.

Guidelines for antibiotics, blanketing (not over an open wound), and pain medication are the same as for lacerations through the skin. Again, tetanus status must be ascertained and antitoxin and/or toxoid administered as indicated.

Laceration with exposed bone:

Any injury involving exposed bone is extremely serious. If infection becomes seated in bone, it can be very difficult, sometimes impossible, to treat, and requires extensive and expensive treatment with intravenous antibiotics. Veterinary attention should be obtained within four hours of the injury to maximize the chances of preventing this complication. Emergency treatment is the same as for other deep lacerations as outlined above, with special care being taken to disturb the injured area as little as possible during cleansing. DO NOT MOVE THE HORSE UNTIL EVALUATED

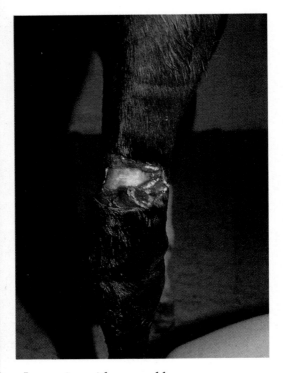

Laceration with exposed bone.

BY A VETERINARIAN, as any bone fragments could move and cause more tissue damage or even sever a nerve or vital blood vessel.

Guidelines for bandaging, antibiotics, blanketing and pain medications are the same as for lacerations involving skin and muscles.

CONTUSIONS—WITH SKIN INTACT * to **

Definition: A contusion is a blunt injury which does not break the skin, but which damages the deep tissues and/or bone. The injured area will show swelling, heat and tenderness.

Treatment: Hose with cold water, 15 to 20 minutes each hour, if possible, or at least three times daily. An alternative is to apply an ice pack under a bandage and leave on for the same amount of time. Severe contusions over the ribs or on the lower legs may have associated fractures. Injury to the abdomen may have caused a defect in the muscles (hernia).

Body wall contusion.

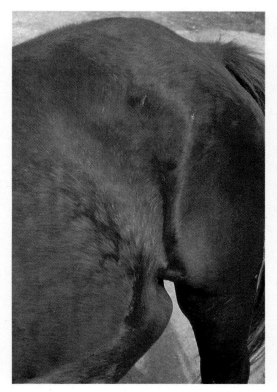

Immediate attention should be sought for swellings that are very large or swellings that increase in size (indicating possible bleeding). If there are any signs of colic after an abdominal injury, or if the horse shows any signs of shock (depression, trembling, sweating) or internal hemorrhage (white gums), get immediate veterinary attention. Record vital signs initially and at hourly intervals until they are stable (three consecutive readings are the same). If the area can be easily bandaged, apply a bandage between hosing or icing treatments.

PUNCTURE WOUNDS **

Definition: A puncture wound is an invasion of skin and deeper tissues with a relatively small entry point. Nails or other sharp objects can cause puncture wounds.

Treatment: If the puncture wound is in the foot, grasp the object firmly and pull straight out. Make a quick sketch of the bottom of the foot with an "X" to mark the spot where the object was located. Heavy bleeding is rare with wounds in the foot (sole or frog area) but some oozing of blood may be seen. The appearance of pus indicates that the wound is old. Clean the foot of debris and manure and soak in hot water with Epsom salts. Administer tetanus toxoid as a booster if the horse has been vaccinated in the past year. Administer both tetanus toxoid and tetanus antitoxin if the vaccination status is unknown or if the horse was last vaccinated over a year ago. Do not administer antibiotics. Call veterinarian to have the wound explored and any other further treatments recommended. If the puncture wound is elsewhere on the body, and the object is small (such as a nail), grasp firmly and pull straight out. With other foreign objects, such as glass or wood, it is best to leave extraction to the veterinarian, as hemorrhage may follow removal of a deeply embedded object. Administer tetanus antitoxin/toxoid as described above. Check with veterinarian before administering antibiotics. Do not flush the depths of a puncture wound prior to veterinary examination—there might be small pieces of debris inside that you could drive in even further.

GUNSHOT WOUNDS ***

Definition: Injuries caused by bullets, pellets, or BBs.

Treatment: Bleeding may be excessive. Uncontrolled bleeding, usually arterial bleeding, is called hemorrhage. Attempt to control as in chapter on Bleeding. When bleeding is controlled, wash gently as described for lacerations. If bleeding does not stop, or requires constant pressure for control, do not attempt to clean the wound. Avoid excessive manipulation of the tissues. Administer tetanus protection and antibiotics as advised under lacerations.

SYMPTOM LIST

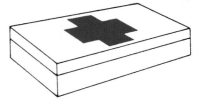

FIRST AID KIT

Clean gauze pads
Quilted leg wraps
Elastic leg wraps
Electrolytes
Belt or tourniquet
Tranquilizer
Blanket
Tetanus toxoid
Tetanus antitoxin
Twitch
Injectable or oral antibiotics

CHAPTER VI

Bleeding

CAUTION: ALWAYS CONTACT THE VETERINARIAN FOR ANY BLEEDING THAT DOES NOT STOP SPONTANEOUSLY WITHIN TEN MINUTES, OR BLEEDING THAT IS NOT FROM AN OBVIOUS CAUSE, SUCH AS A WOUND.

FROM WOUNDS

Oozing *

Oozing is a slow leak or trickling of blood, caused by damage to superficial surfaces.

Treatment: Apply clean gauze or lint-free material to surface of wound. Then apply pressure for three to five minutes. Proceed with treatment as detailed in the chapter on Wounds for the type of injury and area injured.

Venous Bleeding **

Bleeding from veins will vary from minimal to profuse, depending on the size of the blood vessel(s) involved and the area injured. Venous bleeding will stop easily when sufficient pressure is applied. The red color of venous blood is not as bright as the red color of arterial blood.

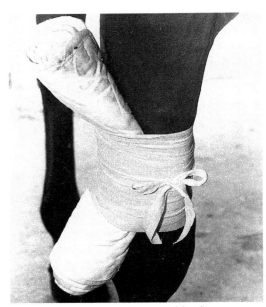

Wrap applying pressure over bleeding area.

Belt used to apply pressure over bleeding point.

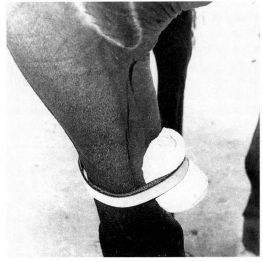

Treatment: Apply clean gauze or lint-free bandage material to surface of wound. Hold in place by hand, or wrap for a minimum of five minutes. If bleeding resumes when pressure is removed, reapply for another five minutes. If bandages soak through quickly, suspect arterial bleeding.

Arterial Bleeding ***

Arterial bleeding is profuse, brisk and bright red. If the artery is located close to the surface, the characteristic pulsations may be seen. With deep arterial bleeding, pulsations may not be obvious, but the wound cavity will fill with blood very quickly. With deep arterial bleeding, tissues surrounding the wound may also swell rapidly.

Treatment: Apply pressure bandaging techniques as described above for venous bleeding. If possible, apply a tourniquet (see photo) with just enough pressure to stop the bleeding. Release tourniquets briefly (for approximately 30 seconds to 60 seconds) every five minutes. If bleeding stops, proceed with wound care. If bleeding does not stop, continue pressure until veterinarian arrives.

FROM NOSE

After Exercise **

Bleeding from the nose may be coming from the upper respiratory tract or from the lungs. The cause may be either the stress of exercise or an underlying disease or infection.

Treatment: Record vital signs every five minutes until stable (no change in three con-

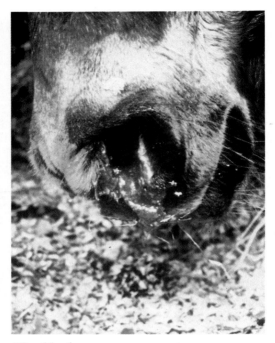

Nosebleed .

secutive readings). If the horse is overheated, sponge with tepid water and apply a light sheet. Keep the horse quiet. If bleeding does not slow significantly in five minutes, or if it is extremely profuse, try elevating the head slightly (you can do this by putting the horse on crossties). But if the horse has trouble breathing or makes choking noises, release the head immediately. DO NOT TRANQUILIZE THE HORSE WITHOUT OBTAINING PERMISSION FROM THE VETERINARIAN FIRST. Do not attempt to pack the nose.

After Injury to the Head ***

Fracture is possible. Since the head area has a rich supply of blood vessels, this type of bleeding could be life-threatening.

Treatment: Record vital signs every five minutes. If horse is trembling and shaky, blanket appropriately according to the weather. Do not raise head or attempt to pack the nose. You may administer pain medication after approval of veterinarian. Do not tranquilize the horse unless recommended by a veterinarian. Place the horse in a quiet stall and avoid undue handling.

Reason Unknown ***

May be caused by an unwitnessed injury, an infection, or a disorder of blood clotting.

Treatment: Record vital signs every five minutes, or until bleeding stops. Note any unusual behavior or unusual color to the mucous membranes. Do not give any medications. Blanket the horse according to the weather, place in a quiet stall, and avoid undue handling.

FROM EARS

After Injury to Head ***

Cause: Probable skull fracture.

Treatment: See chapter on Trauma to Head/ Neck

Reason Unknown **

If the reason for bleeding from ear(s) is unknown, strongly suspect trauma. There may be a deep injury to the ear. Blanket the horse as necessary according to the weather, place in a quiet stall and avoid undue handling. Record vital signs when the injury is first detected, but then do not disturb.

From Wound to Ear *

Treatment: Treat as for any other laceration. If tissue is torn through, avoid excessive pulling. The horse will probably require tranquilization or twitching. If resistance is violent, await arrival of veterinarian.

FROM MOUTH

With Bleeding from Nose ***

Heavy bleeding from throat area or deeper is the probable cause.

Treatment: Record vital signs every five minutes. Blanket according to the weather, and avoid undue disturbance.

With Bleeding from the Nose and With Foaming ***

Cause: Bleeding in the lung and severe respiratory distress. Record vital signs every five minutes. Blanket and avoid disturbing horse.

From Mouth Only **

Cause: Probable injury to gums or tongue. Bleeding from tongue may be very profuse. Do not panic at the amount of blood.

Treatment: Thoroughly rinse mouth with cold water until no grain or hay material is flushed out. Remove hay and grain from stall, but allow access to water (horse may soak or rinse mouth himself). Record vital signs every 10 minutes until stable.

FROM OTHER BODY ORIFICES

From Anus or Vagina Following Breeding ***

Cause: Probable rupture of vagina or rectum.

Treatment: Record vital signs every five minutes. Blanket as necessary if horse shows signs of shock. Administer tetanus toxoid if horse has been vaccinated within the past year; administer both tetanus toxoid and antitoxin if vaccination status is unknown, or if vaccination occurred over a year ago. Administer antibiotics after veterinary approval. Keep animal quiet.

From Anus or Vagina, Not Associated With Breeding ***
Cause: Suspect sadism. Treat as above.

From Vagina Only **
Suspect sadism or accidental injury. Treat as above. (For bloody urine, see chapter on Disorders of Urine/Urination.)

From Anus Only ***
Cause: Probable sadism or freak injury. Tumor a distant possibility. Blood may also be seen with severe intestinal infections when there will be associated diarrhea.

Treatment: If diarrhea is not present, treat as for bleeding following breeding. If diarrhea is present as well, tell veterinarian. Record vital signs every 15 minutes. Offer fresh water as well as electrolyte water. To make electrolyte water, use a commercial equine mix, or add two oz. table salt, one oz. potassium salt (human salt substitute), and one oz. bicarbonate of soda to five gallons of water. Blanket as necessary, and keep horse quiet.

From Penis:

See chapters on Reproductive Organs and Disorders of Urine/Urination.

SYMPTOM LIST

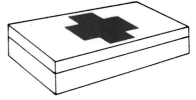

FIRST AID KIT

Mild soap
Silver sulfadiazine cream
Sterile gauze pads
Antibacterial ointment
Antibiotic injection (if ordered by veterinarian based on culture results)
Cold pack
A & D ointment
Zinc oxide

CHAPTER VII

Burns

Burns may be caused by fire, electricity, or chemicals.

SUPERFICIAL BURNS *

Characterized by reddening and swelling of the skin. Animals rarely show blister formation.

Treatment: Clip hair for a generous distance around the burn to better define the extent of the damage. If the burn is caused by chemicals, such as acids, phenols, or strong alkali solutions, hose the area with a strong spray of cold water for at least 15 minutes; then gently clean with mild soap and water. Do not use soap on electrical or flame burns. For other superficial burns, hose the area with cold water for 15 minutes every hour for the first 24 hours, or use a cold pack for same amount of time. Chemical burns should also be treated with cold therapy for 15 minutes out of every hour for the first 24 hours. This may seem like a great deal of work but burns can cause extensive problems that might not show up for several days. If you were the patient, this is the type of intensive therapy you would probably receive.

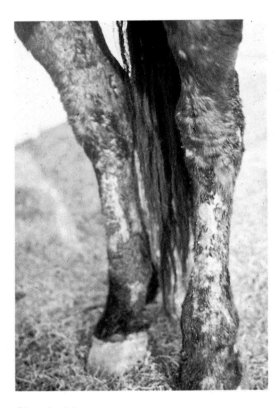

Chemical burn.

DEEP BURNS ***

Definition: A burn which has a break in the skin surface as soon as the injury occurs, or a burn which appears to be intact initially but starts oozing or sloughing off in the first few days.

Treatment: Direct a forceful stream of cool water at the burn for 10 to 15 minutes. Gently but thoroughly clean the area with gentle soap and warm water to remove all dead tissue. Rinse thoroughly with warm water. Allow the burn to dry. Then apply an antibacterial cream such as silver sulfadiazine (treatment of choice). If this is not available, you may use a *light* coating of zinc oxide, A & D cream or ointment, or antibacterial wound cream in the interim. A light bandage of sterile gauze or Telfa may be used. Do not bandage heavily. Clean and dress the area two to three times a day.

Burns .

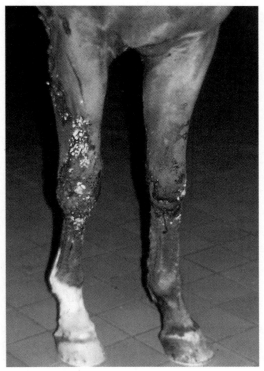

COMPLICATIONS

Scarring: Deep burns may scar badly, particularly if they cover a large area. Skin grafting may be required after the area heals.

Infection: When burns break the skin, infection is always a risk. The best prevention is faithful treatment as above. Always monitor the temperature at least twice daily, or any time the animal appears depressed, until the burn heals. Consult veterinarian before starting any antibiotics.

Shock: Burns which cover a wide surface area may result in the loss of fluids through oozing. This may be sufficient to cause shock. Signs include weakness, trembling, depression, cold ears and extremities, a rapid but weak pulse, and pale mucous membranes with decreased capillary refill time. Monitor for shock by looking for the above signs carefully during the first three days after an extensive burn injury. Record vital signs every hour for the first 24 hours, and four times daily after that or any time the animal seems worse. The horse should continue to drink within his normal range (12 to 20 gallons a day). He may urinate less when in shock. Veterinary coverage is advisable from the start when burns are extensive.

Kidney Damage: Shock may have associated kidney shutdown, so be especially observant of water consumption and urination in animals with extensive burns. Keep track of how many buckets are consumed a day, and how wet the stall is compared to normal. Alert veterinarian immediately if decreased urinary output is suspected. Liver damage may accompany kidney failure.

Lung Damage: Respiratory difficulty may be a late complication of animals trapped in fires or suffering from electrical burns. Observe the horse for increased respiratory rate, noisy breathing, labored breathing, and froth at nose or mouth. Call veterinarian immediately if lung damage is suspected.

SYMPTOM LIST

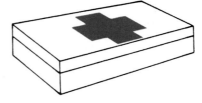

FIRST AID KIT

Acepromazine
Table salt
Peroxide
Dipyrone or Jenotone
Banamine
Rompun
Potassium chloride (salt substitute)
Baking soda or Alka-Seltzer
Disinfectant
Mineral oil
Ivermectin

CHAPTER VIII

Disorders of Eating/ Colic

SALIVATION/DROOLING* to ***

Causes:
1. Choke—blockage of esophagus by bolus of food material
2. Paralysis of throat, as with botulism, lead poisoning or rabies.
3. Tetanus.
4. Irritation of mouth from ingestion of plant or insect.
5. Injury or tumor of mouth or throat.

Diagnosis:

1. *Choke* is most common in older animals during cold weather when water intake may be limited, and in horses fed very coarse hays and/or corn still on the ear or pelleted feeds. Repeated attempts to swallow may be noted. Careful palpation along the neck, in the groove where the jugular vein lies, will often uncover a hard lump which is the blockage.

2. AS IN ALL CASES WHEN *RABIES* IS A POSSIBILITY, THIS SHOULD BE CAREFULLY CONSIDERED BEFORE APPROACHING THE HORSE. IF THE HORSE IS SHOWING ANY SIGNS OF NERVOUS SYSTEM DISTURBANCE, SUCH AS HYPEREXCITABILITY, SENSITIVITY TO

SOUND, OR SEIZURES, DO NOT AT
TEMPT AN EXAMINATION. With *botulism,*
there will also be signs of generalized muscle
weakness and staggering. Movement of the tail
by hand will often show there is little tone or
resistance to manipulation. Anal tone is decreased. With *lead poisoning,* there is also paralysis of the muscles of the larynx, leading to a
dramatic "roaring" noise on respiration with
exercise or excitement. Weakness, staggering
and swollen joints may be present.

**Choke - X-ray of neck showing bulge in
esophagus .**

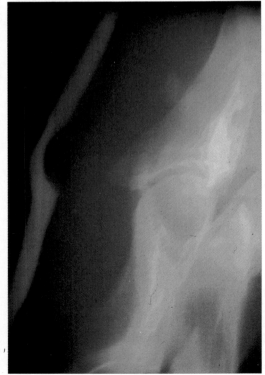

3. *Tetanus* is characterized by inability to open the mouth and a very stiff, "sawhorse" stance with rigidity of the tail.

4,5. *Irritation, injury* or *tumor* of the mouth or throat may be visible on inspection with a flashlight. Pull the horse's tongue to one side to force him to keep his mouth open.

Treatment:

1. *Choke:* Place the horse in a quiet stall. Allow access to water but remove any feed or grain. Obstructions will sometimes pass on their own. Mild tranquilization with Acepromazine is helpful (20 to 30 mg. intramuscularly). If the obstruction is not relieved in the time the tranquilizer has worn off, if there is a foul odor to the breath, or if you are unsure how long the esophagus has been obstructed, get veterinary attention. Delay in relieving the obstruction can result in serious damage to the esophagus and permanent problems. (CAUTION: It is possible for the obstructing lump to disappear from the neck only to become lodged again at the point the esophagus enters the chest. You will not be able to feel it, but the horse will still be unable to move materials into his stomach. Persistence of salivation and refusal to eat or drink will indicate this has happened.)

2,3. Suspected *botulism, lead poisoning* or *tetanus:* If salivation is accompanied by general muscle weakness, decreased anal tone, "roaring," staggering, swollen joints, an inability to open the mouth, or a stiff stance, get immediate veterinary attention. Avoid moving or stimulating the horse in any way.

4. *Mechanical or insect irritation:* If the mouth looks very reddened or an obvious area(s) of

injury or ulceration can be found, flush the
mouth with generous amounts of cold water
(using a hose) to loosen any debris or food in
the mouth and to provide some analgesia.
Allow access to water but no hay or grain for
12 hours. Rinse mouth every two hours with
warm salt water (about 2 tablespoons/quart) or
diluted peroxide solution (about a 10-percent
solution). The mucosa in this area heals
quickly. Offer a mash after about 12 hours but
do not be concerned if horse is not ready to
eat. If horse is not drinking well after 24 hours
and refusing to eat, get veterinary attention for
more complete examination.

5. *Wound or tumor of mouth or throat:* Extensive injuries should receive immediate veterinary attention to prevent the development of
complications. Do not attempt to flush out any
wounds when the horse is not swallowing well,
as the fluid could be inhaled. If breathing
problems develop, see chapter—on Breathing
Problems. Remove all food and water and keep
horse quiet.

FOOD/WATER COMING OUT THE
NOSE * to **

Causes: In foals, this may be a sign of cleft
palate. In adult horses, food may occasionally
come out the nose when eating if the horse
becomes excited and does not swallow properly. Otherwise, problems with the soft palate,
choke, or a paralysis somewhere in the throat
can cause this problem. Temporary difficulties
may develop during severe upper respiratory
infections.

Treatment: Foals should be examined and
treated for cleft palate as soon as possible. The

presence of food along the nasal passages can result in irritation and severe infections. With adults, the occasional appearance of food at the nose when eating is not a cause for much concern unless an abnormal nasal discharge appears. With respiratory infections, the problem may resolve itself as the throat returns to normal. If this is a continuing problem, with large amounts of food or water from the nose and particularly if any abnormal discharge appears, a veterinarian should examine the area with an endoscope to locate the problem and suggest treatment.

COUGHING/CHOKING WHEN EATING * to **

Causes: Coughing or choking during eating may be caused by allergies to the grain or hay, irritation of the throat by infection, a structural abnormality, or paralysis of the throat area.

Treatment: If the problem develops suddenly after switching to a new (possibly dusty or moldy) grain or hay, or if the coughing occurs only when the barn is closed up tightly, suspect an allergy. Go back to feed you know is well-tolerated, or try wetting down the hay or grain slightly before feeding. Problems that develop during a known respiratory infection will usually be self-limiting. You can make things easier by substituting a mash for dry grains during this time and avoiding coarse hays, even if there is no classical "cold" syndrome going on. Two to three-year-old horses may have deep seated infections in the lymphatic tissues of their throats that will often cause this problem.

These horses, as well as any horses with no obvious identifiable cause for the problem, should be examined with an endoscope.

REFUSAL TO EAT/DRINK**

Refusal to eat or drink is a very non-specific sign that something is seriously wrong. It may be caused by an inability to eat or drink (see above sections), or by abdominal pain (see colic, below). However, anything that causes severe pain or makes the horse very ill can result in refusal to eat or drink. You should record the vital signs (temperature, pulse, respiration, as a first step. Think of any recent stresses that could have caused a problem (long shipping, heavy exercise, etc.) and observe for other symptoms that may indicate where the problem lies.

COLIC** to ***

Definition: Colic is a term used to describe abdominal pain of any origin.

Symptoms: The horse with colic will show different signs, depending on the severity and nature of the problem. In mild cases, the horse is depressed, the head is lowered, breathing is somewhat rapid, pulse is normal to slightly elevated, and the horse may look back at his flanks or bite at his flanks. A male may drop his penis. Appetite is poor to absent, although the horse may drink or play. Manure may be absent or abnormal (diarrhea, hard balls with mucus, etc.). As the severity of the problem increases, so does the pain. Horses then begin to show sweating, pawing, pacing, blowing res-

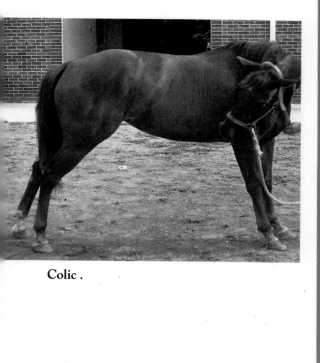

Colic .

Colic .

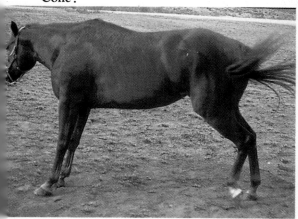

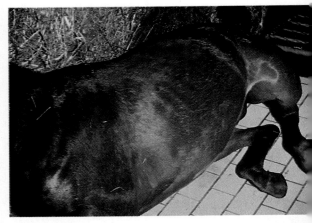

Colic rolling .

pirations, markedly elevated pulse, discolored mucus membranes (bright red or bluish) and want to lie down and roll or thrash.

Causes: Mild cases of colic may be caused by heavy parasite burdens, either in the intestine, stomach or immature forms in the arteries; by old damage from heavy parasite burdens; or by changes in routine, exercise or feed that cause altered eating patterns. Mild colic may stem from impaction, indigestion, diarrhea or spasmodic colic—a condition where a portion of intestine is in spasm, preventing food and gas from traveling on and resulting in distention of the intestine and pain.

Severe cases of colic are usually related to the loss of blood supply to a section of intestine, severe infection/inflammation of the intestine, complete blockage of fecal material and gas from ingestion of foreign material such as rubber fencing, etc., or to twisting or malposition of a section of intestine that also causes a complete blockage. In these cases, the horse also becomes "toxic" as bacterial products are absorbed across the bowel wall. The mucus membranes become bright red or bluish, ears and legs are often cold, founder (terminal), also called (laminitis) may set in as a complication (see chapter on Grain Overload.)

Treatment: With all colic cases, it is important to get organized as a first step. This will give the veterinarian, should he/she be needed, valuable information, and will also serve to give you a clear idea of how the horse is progressing. Do not rely on your memory or vague impressions to make decisions in a colic case.

Purple membranes

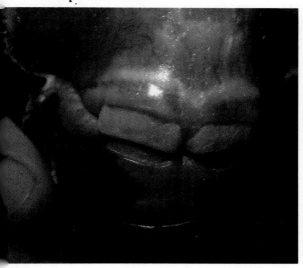

Mild cases of colic often respond to walking or turning out. Walking is advised at first so that you can monitor the horse. Once he has passed gas and manure and seems interested in eating again, it is safe to turn the horse out. Avoid grain for the next 24 hours. Keep hay, salt and water available. Observe the horse frequently over the next 24 hours for signs of recurrence and be aware that colic is something an individual horse may be prone to develop.

Mild cases that do not respond to walking alone will need medication. Dipyrone is a commonly used antispasmodic that can be given intramuscularly at a dose of 10 mg./lb. Allow 15 to 20 minutes to see an effect. This may be repeated in four to six hours. Banamine is also highly recommended for treatment of colic, but, in this author's experience, the onset of relief is prolonged when compared to other agents. Nevertheless, individual horses

Horse with mild colic, showing pawing, slightly elevated tail and standing stretched out.

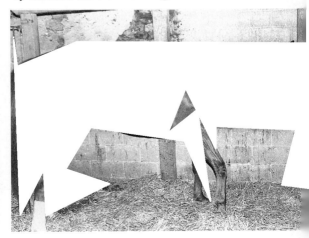

may respond very well. Dose is 0.5 mg./lb. once or twice daily. A less well known anti-spasmodic that works very well, and is this author's drug of choice, is Jenotone. Dosage is 0.25 mg./lb. intramuscularly, up to twice daily. Onset of relief is usually very rapid. This last drug is chemically related to the common tranquilizer, Acepromazine, but does not have the tranquilizing effects. However, if there is no Banamine or Jenotone, you can use Acepromazine in a colic case, giving 25 to 30 mg. intramuscularly. Do not give Acepromazine until the veterinarian has been informed of the horse's vital signs and symptoms (which could indicate impending or present shock) and has approved the use of this drug.

With mild colic cases, it is time to call the veterinarian if:

1. Horse fails to respond to walking or medications.
2. Condition worsens, as indicated by:
   —Increasing pulse and respiration.
   —Worsening pain and agitation.
   —Failure to pass manure for 12 hours or longer. Note if the horse is passing gas or not. Small amounts of liquid may pass a large impaction; do not be fooled by this.
   —Passage of abnormal manure or diarrhea that does not return to normal in one or two bowel movements.
   —Development of signs of laminitis.

As already mentioned, severe pain is the most reliable indicator available to an owner that the horse may have a serious condition. Although horses do vary in their ability to withstand pain, any horse showing violent

pawing, rolling and thrashing needs immediate
veterinary attention. In the interim, proceed
in the same manner as listed for the treatment
of mild colic. However, you should give a tranquilizer as well if the horse is very agitated and
difficult to handle. Rompun at 1 mg./lb. intramuscularly is a good choice. Do not use Acepromazine without prior veterinary approval.
The effect will last one to two hours. Leave
the horse alone after injection (unless he is
rolling and thrashing violently, in which case
you want to try to keep him standing.) Once
the horse has calmed down, proceed as outlined above. If the horse is in a great deal of
distress, it may be best to let him stand quietly
rather than trying to force him to walk, which
could make him attempt to throw himself to
the ground. As a final note on severe colic,
the sudden and unexplained appearance of an
apparent improvement with reduced pain can
be a severe sign. This often signals that a seg-
ment of intestine has ruptured. The apparent
relief is due to reduced pressure along the gut.

DIARRHEA **

Definition: An increase in the frequency of
manure passage or in the amount of manure.
In the horse, diarrhea generally means a
change in manure from well-formed balls to
soft or liquid feces.

Causes: There are many causes of diarrhea.
These include stress, parasites, alteration in
the normal populations of bacteria and other
micro-organisms in the gut, or infections of the
intestines (such as salmonella).

Complications: Laminitis, commonly known as founder, is possible (see chapter Grain Overload). Dehydration.

Treatment: Treat symptoms of diarrhea as described above for mild colic. Avoid alfalfa. Keep fresh water in constant supply. Offer a second bucket containing an electrolyte mixture, either a commercially available premixed powder or one you make up containing:

— 2 oz table salt;
— 1 oz potassium chloride (salt substitute);
— 1 oz baking soda (or 10 plain Alka-Seltzer tablets)

to be added to five gallons of water.

Since there is always the possibility of salmonella infection, which is a hazard to both humans and other animals, a horse with diarrhea should be kept confined to the area where the diarrhea first developed. Wear rubber boots when entering that area and dip them in a disinfection mixture kept in a small tub outside the horse's stall before taking them off. Coveralls for use only in that horse's stall are also a good idea, and be sure to wash your hands immediately after leaving the stall. Do not walk a horse with diarrhea in the barn. Use separate grooming and feeding equipment. Clean that stall last, preferably with a separate pitch fork and rake. If not using separate cleaning tools, disinfect the ones you use when you are finished. Get a sample of the diarrhea in a clean container for your veterinarian to send for cultures.

When to get veterinary attention: With diarrhea, veterinary attention is needed immediately if:

1. Diarrhea is profuse and horse is not drinking or eating.
2. Horse has a temperature over 100° (take temperature three times a day).
3. Diarrhea persists for 24 hours.
4. Signs of colic develop or worsen.
5. Signs of laminitis develop.

CONSTIPATION **

Definition: Failure to pass manure.

Causes: Abnormal intestinal mobility, as with parasite damage; change in diet; inadequate water intake (most common cause); intestinal blockage by sand, rubber fencing or an intestinal "stone" (a hard mass of feces that builds up around a foreign body, known as a fecolith); mechanical blockage such as tumor, abscess or twisted bowel.

Treatment: Horse should be evaluated and treated as described under "Colic." One of the most common causes is inadequate water supply or tainted dirty water that the horse does not drink, so offer plenty of clean water. Try an electrolyte mixture (see above under "Diarrhea"). Exercise is very helpful with simple constipation.

If the horse is eating, offer a warm bran mash with one pint of mineral oil added. To make, add two tablespoons of table salt to three to four scoops of bran. Add boiling water to one inch above the level of the bran. Cover with a cloth and allow to sit until all water is absorbed. Thoroughly mix in 1 pint of mineral oil. You may add ¼ cup (maximum) of corn syrup, molasses or dried molasses powder to improve palatability.

When to get veterinary attention: With constipation, call the veterinarian if:

1. Constipation persists for 12 hours.
2. Signs of colic worsen and do not respond to medication.
3. Signs of laminitis develop.

WORMS IN MANURE *

This is not a true emergency, but many owners panic if they see worms. Obviously, worms in the manure indicate the horse has a parasite problem. Treatment with a good broad-spectrum wormer such as Ivermectin is indicated. It is also common to find worms in the manure after the horse has been given a wormer. This indicates the drug has done its job. If the horse is also showing signs of colic, proceed as above under "Colic."

Date _____

COLIC FLOW SHEET

*TPR = Temperature, Pulse, Respiration

Time	Symptoms	TPR*	(Temp. of) Feet	(Color of) Membranes	Treatment	Comments

SYMPTOM LIST

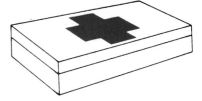

FIRST AID KIT

Baking Soda

Injectable phenylbutazone (for intravenous use only)

Antihistamine solution (intramuscular injection)—A-H Injection

Analgesics for intramuscular injection—Banamine or Torbutrol

Large (at least 20.cc) syringe or dose syringe

CHAPTER IX

Grain Overload (Accidental Overeating)

MILD OVERLOAD

Definition: Horse has received an extra feeding of grain by mistake, or has gotten loose and eaten an amount of grain approximately equal to twice his regular intake.

Symptoms: Horses will vary from no adverse effects at all, to mild depression and transient loss of appetite, to severe problems listed below under heavy overload. Lameness from laminitis (founder) may appear within the first 24 to 48 hours.

Treatment:
1. Withhold all grain for 48 hours.
2. Observe for depression.
3. Observe for abdominal distress (sweating, elevated pulse and respiration, looking at or biting flanks, rolling, pawing, loss of appetite, diarrhea).
4. Check feet hourly for any change in temperature (early laminitis may cause icy cold feet, later stages are hotter than usual to the touch). Note any lameness or reluctance/refusal to move.
5. If signs of abdominal distress develop, begin monitoring every 15 minutes (see colic flow

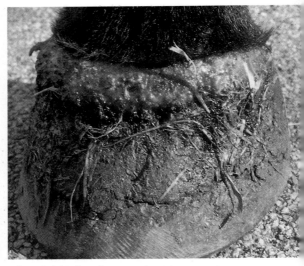

Laminitis, hoof separating .

Founder .

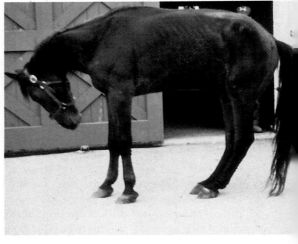

sheet) and consult veterinarian immediately. If emergency visit will be delayed, ask veterinarian about giving five teaspoons of baking soda in 20 cc of water (inject into back of mouth with a syringe) to counteract acidity. NEVER GIVE THIS OR ANY ORAL MEDICATION TO A HORSE IN SEVERE PAIN AND/OR OBVIOUSLY BLOATED. Also see COLIC, page 46.

If temperature changes occur in feet, or if lameness occurs, stand the horse in wet sand or mud to relieve pressure on soles. However, do not force horse to stand or walk. You might consider hosing down the stall if the floor is dirt. Also, the veterinarian may choose to give the horse a nerve block to relieve pain and improve circulation. After this, the horse will usually be comfortable enough to allow the feet to be picked up and packed with mud or poultice. Avoid oral pain medications (e.g. phenylbutazone) as these cause intestinal tract irritation. Intravenous pain medications are appropriate (e.g. 2 grams phenylbutazone). Antihistamine therapy may be helpful (e.g. A-H Injection, 20 cc intramuscularly per 900 to 1,000 pound horse.) Get veterinary attention.

SEVERE OVERLOAD [***]

Definition: Horse with free access to undetermined amount of grain for over 30 minutes or known to have eaten approximately 3 times, or more, than the usual ration.

Symptoms: Depression, rapid breathing, rapid pulse, sweating, pawing, rolling flatulence, loss of appetite, bloating, salivation, later development of diarrhea. (May see all or some of above signs.) Mucous membranes will be bright red to blue-purple in severe cases. Sudden, unexplained lessening of pain, with abnormal mucous membranes and obvious bloating, may signal rupture of stomach.

Complications: Rupture of stomach (see above); laminitis (founder) (see above.)

Treatment:
1. Begin keeping colic flow sheet.
2. Call veterinarian immediately.
3. Remove all hay and water from stall.
4. If veterinarian is not available on immediate emergency basis, obtain veterinarian's approval to give 10 teaspoons baking soda in 20 cc of water. Bloating, an obvious distortion of the flanks (behind the ribs and/or lower belly involving one or both sides). DO NOT GIVE ANYTHING BY MOUTH IN FACE OF SEVERE ABDOMINAL PAIN OR BLOATING. For pain relief, may give Banamine intramuscular or Torbutrol according to manufacturer's recommendations.
5. For laminitis, see above.

SYMPTOM LIST

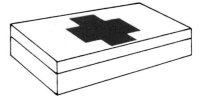

FIRST AID KIT

Large sterile gauze pads
Iodine solution
Peroxide
Rompun   ·
Foot packing or poultice
Alcohol
Mild liniment
Phenylbutazone
Elastic self-adherent wrap, such as
   Vetwrap
Bandages

CHAPTER X

Lameness

DEGREES OF LAMENESS

Lameness is described as 1° (slight), 2° (easily visible), or 3° (total inability or refusal to bear weight). Only 3° lameness can be considered an emergency. This chapter will deal with 2° and 3° lameness.

SYMPTOMS OF LAMENESS

The symptoms of lameness include:
— shortened stride length;
— reluctance to work on circle in the direction of the lame leg;
— resting or pointing the lame leg at rest;
— rough gaits;
— change in performance (e.g. change in jumping style) and/or development of a bad, uncooperative attitude toward work.

There are specific signs that relate to particular areas, such as swinging the leg to the outside with knee pain, but a full description of these is outside the scope of this book and is best left to the veterinarian examining the horse.

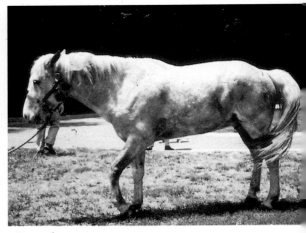

Lame horse .

Favoring left front leg due to pain .

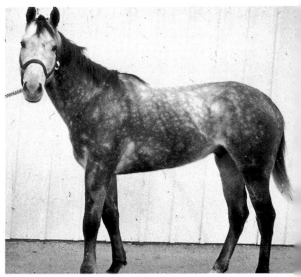

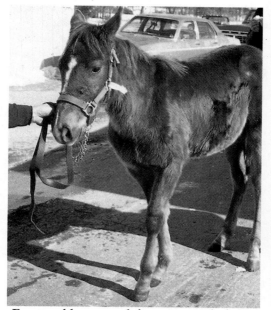

Fractured humerus, left - note weight being taken heavily on opposite front and both hind legs.

DIAGNOSIS

In general, the horse will take shorter strides with his lame leg and come down harder on the opposite leg. The head will drop down when placing weight on the good leg and jerk up on the bad side; this is known as "nodding." Also, when viewed from in front or behind, the horse may move the painful leg in an abnormal manner, swinging it in or out, placing it further under his body when the foot lands, or any other deviation from bringing the leg forward smoothly in a straight line. Lameness is usually more obvious when the horse is worked on hard ground.

Once you feel you have located the sore leg, examination of the leg will help to locate the exact spot of the problem. The three cardinal signs of inflammation are swelling, heat and pain. Begin at the foot and work your way up the leg, comparing the temperature and any amount of swelling with the opposite leg. Pain may be evident when you press the area or, if a joint, when the leg is picked up and the joint flexed. Holding the joint flexed for 30 to 60 seconds and then immediately jogging the horse off will usually cause the lameness to worsen.

TREATMENT

2° Lameness **: Acute injuries, or flare-ups of old problems, may respond to aggressive anti-inflammatory therapy. Hose the affected area with cold water (or soak in a bucket of cold water) for 15 to 20 minutes, three to four times daily. If the problem is in the foot, keep the foot packed with either poultice or a hoof packing. Problems in the fetlocks (ankles), cannon bones, splints or tendons/ligaments below the knees may benefit from wrapping the leg between treatments with water. Massage first with alcohol or a cooling liniment for 5 to 10 minutes. The massage should also be done for higher problems that cannot be wrapped. The above procedures should be done for three days. The horse can also be placed on a three-day course of anti-inflammatory drug therapy with one to two grams of phenylbutazone paste or powder, once or twice daily. On the fourth day, discontinue water therapy and phenylbutazone but continue massage and wrapping. Walking can be started at this time, with a gradual return to work if the horse stays sound.

When to call the veterinarian:
—If lameness worsens or fails to improve after three days of treatment as listed above;
—If lameness returns a day or so after phenylbutazone is stopped.

3° Lameness **: When a horse is refusing to bear weight, or only minimally touching the ground with the involved leg, veterinary attention is indicated on an emergency basis. Do not give large doses of phenylbutazone until the horse has been evaluated by the veterinarian. However, if pain and distress are severe, may give one to two grams of phenylbutazone. The opposite leg, which is taking an increased load, should be wrapped to provide support. If possible, the foot of the "good" leg should be packed with poultice or hoof packing to provide additional support. (Founder in the "good" leg is a common complication of severe lameness.)

FOUNDER/LAMINITIS

See chapter on Grain Overload.

FRACTURE ***

Closed fracture—bone not exposed: Fracture should always be suspected in horses that are 3° lame. In many cases, the fracture will be obvious, with extensive heat, swelling and pain; dangling of the leg below the fracture; abnormal movement of the fractured area. You may

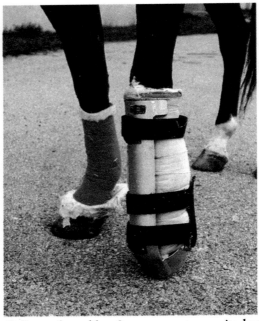

Splint enforced bandage, support opposite leg .

also be able to feel pieces of bone just under the skin.

Treatment: Call for veterinary help immediately. For emergency treatment before the vet arrives, first give a large dose of phenylbutazone (three to four grams) preferably intravenously. If it must be given orally, use a paste preparation or mix the crushed powder with corn syrup or heavy molasses and place on back of tongue. Allow 30 minutes for full analgesic effect. If the animal is extremely agitated, moving around a great deal or generally resisting attempts at treatment, the horse should be tranquilized. However, sedation may worsen unsteadiness in a horse that has sustained the shock of a fracture. Give the horse 10 to 15 minutes in quiet, familiar surroundings before beginning any emergency treatment. The horse should be tranquilized before you try to work on the leg. Rompun is the tranquilizer of choice as it will also give you about 15 minutes of analgesic effect. Give intramuscularly or intravenously at 0.125 mg/lb. dose initially, repeating this in 20 minutes if not adequate. Allow 10 to 15 minutes after giving this drug to evaluate its effect. Sedation may be very profound as the horse has been severely stressed by the severe injury. Be prepared to work on the horse where he is, as moving him is dangerous in terms of the fracture and because of the sedation. To begin, place a good support wrap on the opposite leg (packing the foot will not be possible). Have an assistant gently hold the fractured leg in as close to a normal position as possible, without undue manipulation of the bones. Wrap the involved area with several thick layers of cotton, followed by an elastic, self-adherent wrap, such as Vetwrap. If available, incorporate two pieces of light wood, cork or plastic into the bandage, placing these on top of the cotton and under the elastic wrap. These should extend several inches above and below the fracture site. Use the lightest splint material possible as the weight of this might tend to make the bandage slip down. If it seems safe to walk the horse, proceed very slowly to the closest stall and place in extra bedding. Allow the horse to lie down if he insists on doing so. However, it is best to keep him standing until the veterinarian arrives.

Open fractures: An open fracture is one where bone is protruding through the skin. This is a very serious condition, as infected bone heals poorly and is very difficult to treat.

Treatment: Call the veterinarian and give tranquilizer and pain relief therapy as described above. Cleanse the area by first running cold water over it (direct the water stream above the fracture, not into it) for 15 to 20 minutes. This will control inflammation and pain and help to wash out any debris. Do not attempt to directly clean the fracture area or to touch it in any way. After the hosing, pour peroxide over the wound, again directing it above the fracture and allowing it to run down over it, until the entire surface is "fizzing" white. Leave this on while you gently remove as much dirt and blood surrounding the wound as you can without unduly disturbing the horse. Finally, rinse off the peroxide with cold water. If heavy bleeding is interfering with these procedures, see chapter on Bleeding. Once the wound has been cleaned and bleeding controlled, cover the area with gauze or linen (no cotton or other material with loose fibers) soaked in iodine solution. Carefully proceed with bandaging as described above for closed fractures, making certain the iodine-soaked bandage does not become displaced, exposing the wound to cotton. Keep the horse on his feet until the veterinarian arrives. May give tetanus antitoxin/toxoid if on hand, and antibiotics, but consult with veterinarian first.

SYMPTOM LIST

HEAT STROKE

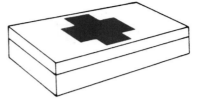

FIRST AID KIT

Ice
Sodium chloride (table salt)
Potassium chloride (salt substitute)
Bicarbonate (baking soda)
Thermometer

CHAPTER XI

Heat Stroke ***

DEFINITION

Heat stroke, heat exhaustion, and sun stroke refer to a disturbance of the heat-regulating mechanisms of the body. This is usually associated with exercise in extreme heat, but may occur in animals left in direct sun with no access to water. An inadequate salt supply may increase the susceptibility to heat stroke, as can repeated exercise (hard work for several days in a row) in hot weather or the use of diuretics.

SYMPTOMS

Symptoms include muscular cramping, profound weakness or collapse, muscle tremors, profuse sweating, rapid breathing, and a rapid pulse. Working animals may simply refuse to go further and drop in their tracks. Rectal body temperature may be greatly elevated (up to 109°F or greater). Mucous membranes are brick red. Staring and unresponsiveness may also occur.

TREATMENT

The primary goal of treatment must be to lower body temperature. Hose the animal with cold water. Place ice packs around the body. The rectum may be packed with cracked ice, but this removes the possibility of monitoring temperature to determine effectiveness of therapy. There is the possibility of causing damage to the rectum, resulting in life-threatening infection in the abdomen. In general, while ice in the rectum is highly effective, its use should be withheld for cases where the temperature remains extremely high despite other measures. (You may try positioning the thermometer for an oral reading if the animal is not objecting; the temperature will be at least one degree lower than rectal.) Veterinary aid should be obtained as quickly as possible to administer intravenous fluids. Animals willing to drink should be offered their choice of fresh water and electrolyte water. (Use a commercial mix or add one oz. table salt, one oz. salt substitute [potassium chloride] and five tablespoons of baking soda to five gallons of water.) Increase the table salt to two oz. if baking soda is not available. Horses that are willing to stand and move should be transported to a cool and shady area. Prostrate horses should not be moved. A temporary shade should be erected over them, with only a top so the air can circulate.

SYMPTOM LIST

FIRST AID KIT

Sodium chloride
Potassium chloride
Baking soda
Acepromazine
Phenylbutazone
Banamine

CHAPTER XII

Exercise-Related Problems

EXHAUSTION/HEAT PROSTRATION **

Symptoms: Marked depression after exercise, loss of appetite, refusal to drink, continued sweating, elevated pulse, temperature and respiratory rates beyond 15 to 20 minutes post-exercise.

Cause: Overwork.

Treatment: See chapter on Heat Stroke. Make certain horse has free access to water and salt after being cooled out.

"THUMPS" **

Definition: "Thumps" is a condition of severe electrolyte disturbances in which the diaphragm is stimulated to move synchronously with the heart beat.

Symptoms: A jerking to heavy thumping movement behind the last rib, in the flank, occurring in a horse with one or more symptoms of overwork.

Treatment: See chapter on Heat Stroke. Calcium, potassium and magnesium are the primary electrolyte disturbances responsible for the problem, together with dehydration and alterations in pH of the blood and chloride content. Horses that do not respond after eating and drinking and/or within two to three hours, will require intravenous specialized electrolyte mixtures given by the veterinarian.

TYING-UP **

Definition: Severe and persistent muscular cramping which occurs during or immediately after exercise or some excitement.

Symptoms: Extreme anxiety and/or depression; elevated pulse and respiratory rates (secondary to pain); reluctance or refusal to move; rigid stance; rock-hard musculature, primarily in the large muscles of the hindquarters; dark urine.

Tying-up.

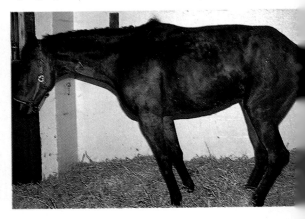

What to do: Move the horse as little as possible. Forced exercise—even walking—can cause more muscle breakdown. If the horse has been competing or exercising some distance from the barn, transport by trailer. If the weather is cool, blanket the horse and protect from drafts. Offer both fresh and electrolyte water (see chapter on Heat Stroke). Give 20 to 30 mg. of Acepromazine tranquilizer. Give two to three grams of phenylbutazone paste or slurry (or intravenous injection) or 500 mg. of Banamine for pain and inflammation. Observe the urine carefully. Dark urine indicates the presence of muscle pigment, a severe sign. If urine color is not clear by the second time the horse urinates, get immediate veterinary attention, as the muscle pigment can plug the kidneys and cause renal failure.

When to call the veterinarian:
1. If urine remains dark on two separate urinations.
2. If condition is not improved after drug therapy recommended above.
3. If horse is refusing all water for more than one hour.

Conditions that may be confused with tying-up:
1. Laminitis.
2. Coffin-bone fractures.
3. Severe chest pain.
4. Severe abdominal pain.
5. Tetanus.

All of the above can cause the horse to be reluctant to move, stand stiffly, and shift his weight to the hindquarters—making the hind-end muscles tense up.

SYMPTOM LIST

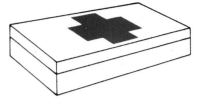

FIRST AID KIT

Thermometer
Vicks
Blanket
Phenylbutazone
Cough suppressant recommended by veterinarian
Vaporizer
Expectorant recommended by veterinarian (e.g. sodium iodide powder)
Vaseline
Scalpel and emergency breathing tube (for tracheotomy)
Gauze pads
Antibiotics
Tranquilizer
Tetanus antitoxin and toxoid

CHAPTER XIII

Breathing Problems

RAPID RESPIRATION* to ***

Definition: Respiratory rate of over 15 breaths per minute is rapid.

Nonspecific causes: Pain, fear, exercise.

Respiratory causes: Infection of the lungs or chest (check for one or more of the respiratory symptoms listed below in this chapter). Allergy.

Treatment: Count and write down the number of breaths per minute. Blanket the horse if weather dictates, and keep out of drafts. Check for and write down any other symptoms. Take temperature. Contact veterinarian with above information and follow instructions. Get emergency attention if breathing is obviously difficult and horse is agitated or depressed.

NOISY RESPIRATION *to ***

Definition: Any noise that occurs with breathing (normal respiration is silent).

Nonspecific causes: Pain may cause the horse to make blowing or grunting noises.

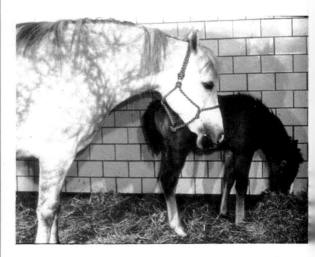

Respiratory distress in foal.

Respiratory causes: Anatomical abnormalities along the upper airways (nose and throat) can block the normal flow of air and cause the horse to make a noise. Swelling anywhere along the upper airways or windpipe does the same thing (e.g. from trauma, infection or allergic reactions). Infections in the lungs may cause excessive secretions that obstruct air flow.

Types of Noises:
Blowing: Forceful, hard breathing, as occurs after exercise or if horse is in pain.
Wheezing: High-pitched squeaking noises which are usually most obvious when the horse is breathing out.
Whistling: High-pitched fluttering or flute-like noises, usually more obvious during one phase of respiration (i.e. either when breathing out or breathing in).

Rattling: Coarse, wet or dry noises that are heard throughout respiration, associated with collection of fluid or mucus along the respiratory tract.

CAUSES AND WHAT TO DO

Blowing: Blowing after exercise is normal. Depending on the exercise, it lasts from a few minutes to 15–20 minutes. If horse does not recover after 20 minutes, take temperature. Walk horse to check for signs of lameness or reluctance to move that might indicate a source of pain. If other abnormalities are found, see appropriate sections of this book. If horse is overheated (temperature over 100° after 20 minutes), sponge or hose with tepid water. If no other cause is found, schedule veterinary examination to check for breathing problems.

If the horse is blowing without relation to exercise, moderate to severe pain is usually the cause. Fever may also cause blowing, so take temperature. Try to determine cause of pain by walking horse and checking stall for anything abnormal (e.g. change in or lack of manure). Seek emergency attention and treatment.

Wheezing: Wheezing may be caused by allergic/asthma type reactions ("heaves") or accumulation of dry mucus in the lungs during or after a respiratory infection. Exercise may worsen wheezing to the point at which it is audible without a stethoscope. If there is no history of infections, the horse may be relieved by taking him outside, since most irritants are found in the barn, hay and straw. If the wheezing does not stop, or if the horse is depressed and working very hard to breath, emergency attention is needed. Otherwise, schedule a visit for evaluation and recommendations for medication and management.

Whistling: Whistling noises associated with exercise, excitement or any elevated breathing rate usually signal a structural problem in the upper airways (e.g. "roaring", growths, cysts or other problems). Noise will abate if the horse is kept quiet, but diagnosis and treatment will eventually be necessary. If whistling appears suddenly, is not associated with exercise, and does not go away when horse is kept quiet, seek emergency attention. Cause is likely to be a sudden blockage to breathing from an abscess or tumor or collection of infection somewhere. Check throat area (between jaw bones) for swelling or drainage of pus likely to be "Strangles" infection. Take temperature and get immediate attention.

Rattling: Rattling noises, as already stated, accompany collections of fluid or mucus along the respiratory tract. Take temperature and note any other symptoms (e.g. cough or nasal discharge). Keep horse quiet and warm. Liberal use of Vicks and a vaporizer will help to loosen the secretions. Do not start antibiotics without consulting veterinarian (these will interfere with any necessary cultures). For temperature over 100°, depression, loss of appetite or obvious difficulty in breathing, seek emergency attention.

FLARED NOSTRILS **

Definition: Nostrils blown wide open with each breath, usually accompanied by blowing (see above).

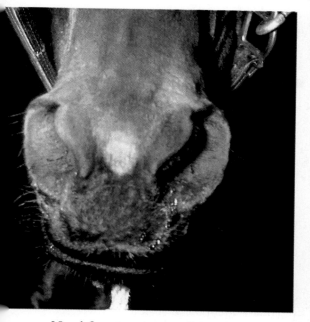

Nasal flare (respiratory distress).

Causes: Flaring is associated with hard breathing of any cause. It is a sign that the horse is working hard to get air. This is normal for a short period after exercise, but at other times indicates the horse has a problem with getting enough air. On occasion, the hard breathing associated with severe pain will also cause flaring.

Treatment: Flaring not associated with exercise indicates the horse is not getting sufficient air. Take temperature, avoid all stress (do not move the horse), protect from cold and drafts, record any other symptoms, and get emergency attention.

COUGH* to ***

CAUSES AND WHAT TO DO

Cough is caused by any irritation (infection or otherwise) along the respiratory tract.

Dry Cough: Caused by early viral infections or irritation from dust/allergens. Take temperature three times daily. If fever is present, suspect probable early viral infection. Watch for nasal discharge (clear with uncomplicated virus, yellow or grey with bacterial infection). Avoid cold and drafts, and keep horse in stall until temperature is normal for 24 hours. Encourage eating with high-quality hay and mashes. Avoid all medications unless absolutely necessary. With constant cough, may give an over-the-counter equine cough medicine for a day or two. If cough persists, seek veterinary attention. If high fever (over 100°) is present on two consecutive readings, may give one to two grams phenylbutazone once a day, but for not more than two days. If fever persists at high levels, if cough is severe, if there is a white-yellow or grey discharge, or if any other respiratory symptoms listed in this chapter are severe, get veterinary attention. DO NOT GIVE ANTIBIOTICS without consulting veterinarian. The horse and his equipment should be isolated as well as possible from other animals, since respiratory infections are highly contagious.

If there is no fever or other sign of infection, the probable cause of a dry cough is allergy ("heaves"). For a severe attack, get immediate attention. Otherwise, put the horse outside, and feed only clean, dust-free hay and grain. Consult veterinarian if problem persists.

Moist Cough: A wet cough is almost always associated with respiratory infection—either a complication of viral infection or following allergic irritation. A cough no longer moist could be pneumonia. Nasal discharge may not be visible if the horse is swallowing his secretions. Avoid cold and drafts. No exercise. Keep secretions loose with vaporizer and Vicks. If these measures do not provide relief in a day, or if horse is obviously not getting any better, seek veterinary attention. DO NOT GIVE ANTIBIOTICS without consulting veterinarian. Do not give cough suppressants when a moist cough is present.

NASAL DISCHARGE* to.***

Definition: Fluid from the nostrils.

Causes: Mechanical irritation or infection. Cold alone causes some horses to have a con-

Pus from one side of nose (gutteral pouch).

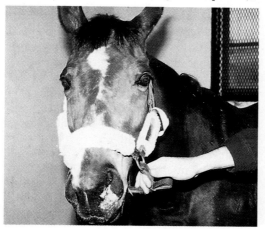

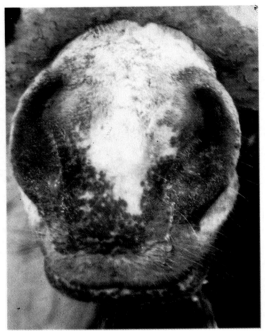

Pus from nose (Sinusitis) .

stant clear discharge. A clear to frothy-white discharge is also common after exercise and not a cause for concern. Danger signs include: heavy discharge associated with abnormal breathing; yellowish, greyish, thick discharge; and discharge from one side only (caused by infection or structural problem in the nasal passages, sinuses or throat). Seek immediate attention if horse is having trouble breathing. Schedule an examination to find the cause if horse is not in immediate distress. Take temperature two to three times daily. Record all other symptoms. DO NOT GIVE ANTIBIOTICS without veterinary approval. Keep nostrils wiped clean and coated with Vaseline to avoid skin irritation.

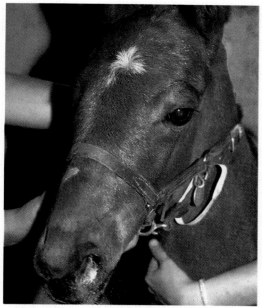

Cleft palate with nasal discharge

Heavy nasal discharge

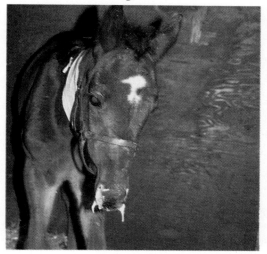

REDUCING RISK OF
RESPIRATORY INFECTIONS

1. Vaccinate all horses well in advance of cold weather. Vaccinate year-round for horses that travel extensively and are exposed to outside horses.

2. During an outbreak, keep all obviously infected horses away from direct contact with well horses. Use separate buckets, blankets, etc.. Wash hands between working with horses. Ventilate barn well but avoid direct drafts. Take temperatures twice daily of horses that appear well. Immediately remove horses that develop temperature elevation or other symptoms from contact with well horses. If possible, keep well horses in another building or even outside. May vaccinate horses that remain well if they have been without temperature elevation or other symptoms for seven days after the start of the outbreak. (If the horse is incubating the disease, vaccination may result in illness.)

BLEEDING FROM NOSE

See Chapter on Bleeding.

TRAUMA TO
NECK/THROAT ** to ***

An injury to the neck or throat area should be evaluated to determine if it needs veterinary attention (see chapter on wounds).

EMERGENCY TRACHEOTOMY

If the horse is making abnormal breathing sounds, get veterinary help immediately. If the horse becomes violent, do not attempt restraint—it will be impossible. However, once he has collapsed (from lack of oxygen), immediately spread open the edges of the wound, locate the windpipe or throat area and try to locate a hole. Spread this open as widely as possible and remove any muscle or other tissue that might be in the way. Ideally, you will need to place something in the hole to keep it open. The outside cylinder of a 20 cc syringe is the perfect size for this. It should be positioned perpendicular to the windpipe or top of the throat so that it does not fall down into the windpipe.

All of this may sound like more than you can possibly do. However, once the horse is down and has stopped struggling, you will be free to work. Also, after he has regained consciousness, he will be far less likely to struggle. Someone should be sitting on the horse's head until he is fully conscious. When he is getting up, stay close to the head at all times to keep the syringe in place until help arrives.

If the horse has suffered a severe blow or crushing type injury to the throat or neck area and is having trouble breathing, even though the skin is not broken, he has crushed or fractured a part of his respiratory tract, or is having his air choked off by severe swelling or bleeding into the tissues. Call for emergency attention and keep the horse as quiet as possible. NEVER TRANQUILIZE A HORSE HAVING BREATHING PROBLEMS—this may depress breathing further. If air becomes blocked completely and the horse collapses, once he is unconscious you must place an airway, as described above for open wounds, after making an incision through the skin over the

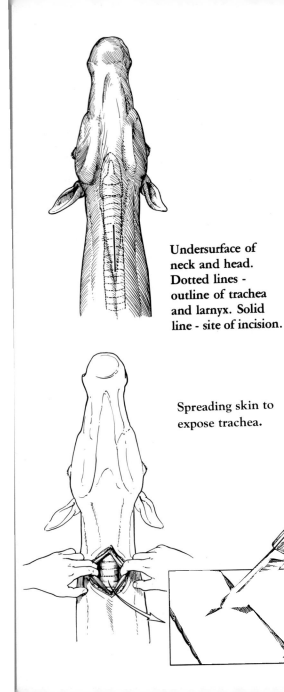

Undersurface of neck and head. Dotted lines - outline of trachea and larnyx. Solid line - site of incision.

Spreading skin to expose trachea.

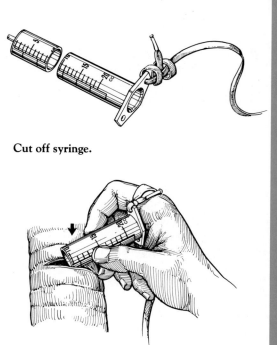

Cut off syringe.

Cut off syringe, as described in text, inserted in tracheal incision.

Syringe, tied in place around neck.

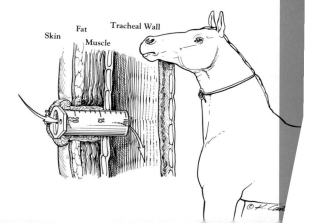

Skin   Fat   Tracheal Wall   Muscle

trachea. Feel for the windpipe through the skin, about 4 to 5 inches below throat level. Feel for the tracheal rings, which feel like ridges. Pull the skin tight over the trachea with one hand and cut boldly all the way through the skin and underlying tissues. Don't worry about bleeding at this point. Don't worry about cutting into the trachea. It is very tough and hard to enter. When you can feel the trachea directly, punch into it with the point of your knife then enlarge the hole just enough to allow the syringe to fit through snugly. Quickly check that air is moving through the syringe and pack the area between the skin edges and the syringe tightly with gauze sponges or even paper towels if nothing else is available (do not use cotton as it will get into the open wound and leave fibers). The horse will arouse quickly once he is getting air again.

This procedure is definitely not something that should be attempted by anyone who is at all uneasy at the idea, as you must work quickly and surely. This is one procedure that is definitely best discussed in advance with your veterinarian. When he is visiting, have him show you how to proceed, should you need to perform a tracheotomy, where to go in, etc., and ask him to answer any questions you may have.

TRAUMA TO CHEST **

Open wounds/Puncture wounds: Wounds which penetrate through the skin and muscle of the chest wall allow air to enter the chest cavity, and this causes collapse of the lung. You should not attempt to treat any injury that looks as if it may have penetrated into the chest. Apply pressure if the wound is bleeding. Otherwise, place the horse in a quiet stall and get immediate veterinary attention. Another complication of penetrating chest wounds may be damage to the lung tissue, which results in air escaping out of the lung. This will make its way into the chest cavity and may spread into the tissues of the wound, causing them to swell. Air in the tissues is termed subcutaneous emphysema and can be recognized by a characteristic crackly feeling to the involved areas, similar to the feel of packing materials that are made up of tiny plastic air bubbles. Again, emergency veterinary attention is needed. Tetanus antitoxin and toxoid and antibiotics may be given, but check with the veterinarian before giving any antibiotic.

Penetrating wound on chest.

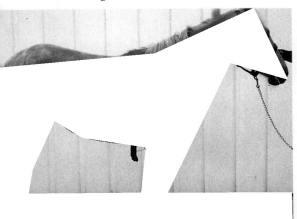

Blunt Trauma to Chest Wall: Heavy blows or bumps to the chest wall can result in contusion of the lung, with possible bleeding into the chest cavity and/or broken ribs. The horse will show depression, reluctance to move and a very shallow breathing pattern. If the horse is in severe distress—refusing to eat or drink, with rapid and difficult breathing—emergency veterinary attention is in order. With less severe signs, a trial of three grams of phenylbutazone may be given to determine the contribution of pain to his symptoms. If the horse shows obvious relief after phenylbutazone, trauma to the muscles/ bones of the chest wall is probably the major problem. Keep him on phenylbutazone at one to two grams daily. If there is no significant improvement, or if the condition worsens or fever develops, seek veterinary attention.

COLLAPSE

SYMPTOM LIST

CHAPTER XIV

Collapse

NOTE: This chapter deals with loss of consciousness/seizure activity which occurs unexpectedly, for no apparent reason. For collapse with an obvious cause—e.g. exhaustion, heat prostration, breathing emergency—see the appropriate specific section.

SYMPTOMS

Loss of consciousness/seizure activity may occur unexpectedly or be preceded by behaviour changes. It is important to note all surrounding events, before, during, and after the episode, to aid in diagnosis and proper treatment. Behavior changes preceding loss of consciousness or a seizure may range from depression or blank staring to agitation and hypersensitivity to stimuli such as light, touch or sounds. Loss of consciousness may last for seconds to minutes, with the horse lying quietly or showing twitching and/or thrashing movements (seizure activity—see below). After regaining consciousness, the horse may be completely normal or may seem dazed, depressed or confused.

Colic.

LOSS OF CONSCIOUSNESS**

Definition: Losing consciousness, or "passing out."

Possible Causes: Loss of consciousness could be caused by cardiac problems, could be a type of seizure, or could be related to a lesion in the brain following trauma. Cardiac problems or a specific disorder of the brain called narcolepsy are the most likely causes of altered consciousness without seizure movements. The horse may collapse entirely or may seem to suddenly fall asleep and buckle at the knees. With cardiac causes, exercise may or may not precipitate the attack, depending on the nature of the specific disorder underlying the problem. With narcolepsy there will usually be some specific stimulus that triggers the attack—eating, leading the horse, stroking the horse a particular way, etc.

Treatment: No specific emergency treatment is necessary. In terms of prevention, if it is possible to identify a precipitating cause, that should obviously be avoided. There is a good chance that drug therapy will be helpful but a complete veterinary examination must first determine the cause. A detailed description of the event will aid this diagnosis.

SEIZURES/"FITS"**

Symptoms: Seizure activity is an abnormal firing of nerve cells in the brain which results in loss of consciousness and any of the following signs: twitching, jerking, limb movement, neck stiffness, movements of eyes and lips, urination, defecation, salivation, sweating. Seizures may be separated by minutes, hours, days, months or even years.

Causes: Seizures (epilepsy) may be a congenital problem (epilepsy); secondary to damage from decreased blood supply, infection, trauma or tumor; related to liver failure; or may appear as the predominant symptom of rabies.

Treatment: No attempt should be made to restrain or "wake up" a horse having a seizure. The danger to you is too great. After the seizure is over, remove any buckets from the stall, darken the stall and keep all stimulation of any kind to an absolute minimum. Precise recording of the seizure activity is critical to diagnosis. Note particularly if the abnormal movements occurred on both sides of the body, if all parts of the body or only some were involved, or if the animal lost urine or feces during the seizure. Because of the danger that the seizure activity could be a manifestation of rabies, extreme caution should be used if there is even the remotest chance the horse has been exposed to a rabid animal. Do not attempt to treat any self-inflicted injuries or to comfort/reassure the horse, since there is no way to predict whether another seizure is going to occur. Veterinary attention will be needed to treat the current episode, determine the cause of the seizure, and institute the correct drug therapy.

DISORDERS OF BALANCE, COORDINATION, PERSONALITY

SYMPTOM LIST

CHAPTER XV

Disorders of Balance, Coordination, Personality

SYMPTOMS OF NEUROLOGICAL DISEASE

Symptoms of acute neurological disease are generally very dramatic. The horse may show any of the below signs, in any combination:

— staggering
— loss of coordination
— dragging of toes
— falling to the side
— inability to back up
— falling
— personality changes
  — aggression
  — marked depression
  — stupor
  — staring
  — panic
— apparent blindness
— running into walls
— violent thrashing
— twitching of face or body
— loss of consciousness
— seizures.

CAUSES

The specialty of neurology, and details of all the possible causes for the above symptoms, is too extensive to be appropriate for a first aid book. However, you should know enough about the possible causes to recognize what could be producing these symptoms in your horse. Some general categories are given below.

Head tilt, encephalitis (brain inflammation).

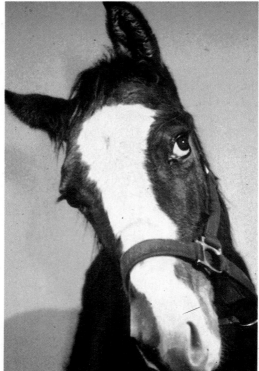

—Infections: Viral, bacterial, fungal or protozoal infections can all cause central nervous system disease. The primary symptoms are usually related to loss of balance and coordination, rather than personality changes or seizures. Your vet will need to know the horse's vaccination history and any history of infectious diseases in the past, particularly respiratory infections (even if mild) or strangles.

—Feed-related: Moldy corn contains a toxin that destroys brain tissue. If you feed corn in any form, including a sweet feed or pellet with corn in it, this could be the source.

—Plant poisoning: There are several plants that can cause neurological problems. Many of these do so by causing liver damage, which allows poisons which affect the brain to build up in the body. Violent periods, interspersed with periods of marked depression, are the rule here. The horse may injure himself badly during the violent episodes. In addition, the mucous membranes will be yellow-orange in color. Urine will be dark.

—Lead poisoning, tetanus, botulism and rabies are all associated with varying degrees of neurological dysfunction. Loss of swallowing ability and heavy salivation are early symptoms of this.

—Causes within the brain itself may include tumors, injury secondary to trauma or interference with the normal blood supply.

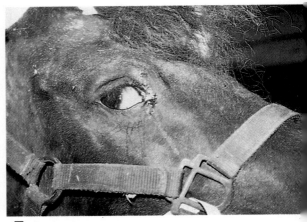

Tetanus eye .

Tetanus .

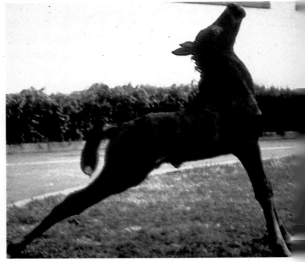

EMERGENCY TREATMENT

The sudden onset of neurological signs is an emergency condition that calls for prompt veterinary attention, rapid diagnosis and specific treatment if there is to be any hope of recovery. Put the horse in as large a stall as possible and remove all projections from the walls, including buckets. Bedding should be deep in case of falls. No treatment should be given before the vet arrives. If rabies is at all possible, stay away from the horse.

If signs suggesting liver disease are present, as above, do not use any field that the horse may have been turned out in for other horses until a plant expert can check it out. If your feed contains any corn, stop using it and save a sample for analysis. It is possible for only one horse to show signs, even if all are getting the same feed.

SYMPTOM LIST

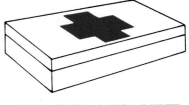

FIRST AID KIT

Phenylbutazone tablets
Blanket
Acepromazine tranquilizer injection

CHAPTER XVI

Trauma to the Head and Neck

BLOWS TO THE HEAD

Causes: Blows to the head may be inflicted by humans, or may be accidental, as when a horse rears and strikes his head.

Consequences: The consequences of a severe blow to the head depend upon the area injured. Blows below the level of the eyes may injure facial bones, sinuses or jaw. Injury to eye area may damage eye itself (see eye chapter) or the orbit (bony socket of the eye). Blows higher on the head may injure the skull and/or brain and spinal cord.

Sinus injury/fracture *to***

Symptoms: Deformity of face in area of blow, bleeding from nostril(s), noisy respiration, or decreased air flow from nostril(s).

Complications: Infection is likely. Pus-like drainage may begin as soon as 24 to 48 hours after the injury. Appearance of pus at the nostrils may be delayed if drainage is blocked by the injury. Observe for increased facial swelling.

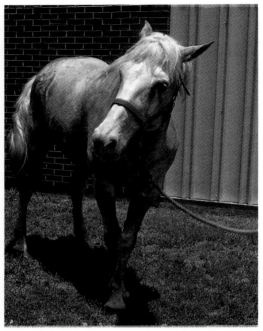

Spinal cord disease with difficulty balancing.

Nosebleed.

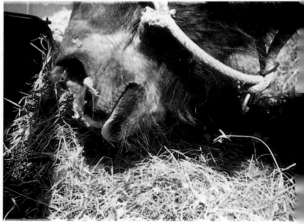

Treatment:

1. Nosebleed—see chapter on Bleeding. May tranquilize horse lightly if bleeding is not profuse (get veterinary approval first).

2. Remove halter if it is tight or putting direct pressure on injured area. Pad the halter well before replacing.

3. Observe for signs of severe respiratory distress, i.e. depression, flared nostrils, or a respiratory rate over 25 at rest.

4. May give one to three grams of phenylbutazone for pain.

5. Monitor temperature twice daily for seven days. Prophylactic antibiotic coverage (e.g. penicillin) may be started on approval of veterinarian.

6. Get veterinary attention for any of the following:

   —Obvious deformity/swelling;
   —Noisy respiration;
   —Decreased air flow from one or both nostrils;
   —Heavy or persistent bleeding;
   —Temperature elevation to 100°F or greater on two or more consecutive readings;
   —Pus or foul odor from nostrils;
   —Refusal to eat or drink within 12 hours of injury;
   —Difficulty with chewing or swallowing food/water.

Fractured jaw **

Symptoms: Swelling in area of jaw "clicking" noise on jaw movement, pain on pressure over jaw, refusal or reluctance to eat or drink.

Treatment: Remove halter if it is putting pressure on injured area. Pad the halter well before replacing. May give one to three grams of phenylbutazone as above for pain. Call veterinarian immediately if horse is not eating or drinking. Will need x-rays to determine exact treatment needed.

Injury to area of eye ***

Symptoms: See eye chapter for injuries to the eye itself. Extreme pain, swelling or obvious deformity, bulging of eye, apparent blindness on affected side may all indicate injury to the structures around the eye.

Treatment: Call veterinarian immediately if any of the above symptoms are present. Delay in treatment could result in blindness. May give one to three grams of phenylbutazone to control pain.

Trauma to skull/brain/spinal cord ***

Symptoms: Symptoms of skull fracture include any obvious deformity of the injured area, marked swelling, or neurological signs indicating concussion or brain hemorrhage. Neurological signs include: head held tilted; staggering; swaying; pupils of unequal size; pupils with decreased or no reaction to light; and blood or clear fluid draining from ear. Injuries to spinal cord high in the neck may cause above signs plus refusal to turn or bend neck, or sudden paralysis, or sudden death from paralysis of muscles of respiration,

Treatment:
1. Do not attempt to move animal.
2. May tranquilize lightly if horse is agitated or struggling. Try to avoid this.
3. Give 2 to 3 grams of phenylbutazone to control pain and help with inflammation.
4. Blanket (heaviness according to weather) as general supportive care against shock.
5. Get immediate veterinary attention.

FLIPPING OVER BACKWARDS***

Brain and Spinal Cord
Symptoms: Injury to skull, brain, or spinal cord, as described above, is very likely.

Treatment: Do not force horse to stand. Quietly remove any restricting equipment (side reins, etc.) and stand back. If horse is not up in a few minutes and/or if showing any of the signs listed under trauma to skull/brain/spinal cord, treat as above.

Other fractures
Note: Horses which go over backwards may also suffer fractures of the lower spine (back and rump), pelvis, ribs, or other bones. Check carefully over the next few days for any areas of tenderness or swelling. Extreme muscular tenderness/spasm along the back may indicate a fracture in that area. Rapid, shallow respiration, reluctance to move, or extreme resentment of girth may indicate rib fracture. Contact veterinarian if severe injury of this type is suspected. May control pain with phenylbutazone, one to three grams once or twice daily.

SYMPTOM LIST

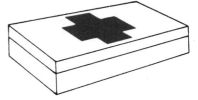

FIRST AID KIT

Cotton swabs (Q-Tips)
Rompun tranquilizer injection
Fly repellant
Antibiotic ophthalmic ointment or drops
  (no steroids added)
Atropine ophthalmic ointment or drops
Cold compresses
Twitch

CHAPTER XVII

Eyes

SWOLLEN EYE**

Possible Causes: Insect sting, blow to the eye, foreign material under eyelids, or injury to eyelids or eye itself.

Treatment:
1. Restrain horse (twitch may be needed).
2. Open eye to check for obvious damage to eye itself.
3. Pull down lower eyelid to look for dirt, plant material, or other matter. If foreign matter is identified on inner surface of eyelids, you may attempt removal by touching this gently with a dry cotton swab. Do *not* attempt removal of any material which is on the eye itself. Do not attempt removal if horse is not well restrained.
4. Note any swelling or redness of inner surfaces of eyelids and report this to veterinarian.
5. Place horse in dark, quiet stall.
6. Apply cold moist compresses to the closed eye every 15 to 20 minutes for five minutes at a time until the veterinarian arrives. You may be able to bandage these in place, using an elastic leg wrap looped around the sides of a halter and behind the ears.

TEARING *to**

Possible Causes: Tearing may accompany any other injury to the eyelid or eye, or may be caused by a blocked tear duct.

Treatment:
1. Try to determine if the eyes or eyelid are injured. If there is no obvious injury—if the eyes are held wide open and horse does not object to light—problem is probably a blocked tear duct. Veterinarian will have to insert a small tube and flush this clear.
2. If there is an injury to the eyelid or eye itself, follow instructions elsewhere in this chapter.

INABILITY TO OPEN EYELIDS***

Possible Causes: Damage to facial nerve which innervates the muscles controlling eyelid movement. Brain tumor or infection may involve upper and/or lower eyelid.

Treatment:
1. Differentiate inability from refusal to open eyelids by noting that eyelids are droopy and horse shows little resistance to having eyelids moved manually. There may also be associated paralysis of ear, nostril, or lip on the same side of the face.
2. If the eye is only partially closed, it may be very dry and/or injured.
3. Place the horse in dark stall.
4. Remove halter, particularly if tight, as this may be placing pressure on the facial nerve.
5. Contact veterinarian.

REFUSAL TO OPEN EYELIDS **
to ***

Possible Causes: Refusal to open eyelids indicates eye pain. This may be due to an injury to the eye or eyelids, or to a disease of the eye such as periodic ophthalmia (moon blindness).

Treatment: Same as for swollen eye.

LACERATION TO EYELIDS ***

Possible Causes: Direct trauma to eye.

Treatment:
1. Try to determine if the eye itself is also injured. However, do not manipulate the injured eyelid.
2. Follow the same treatment as for swollen eye.

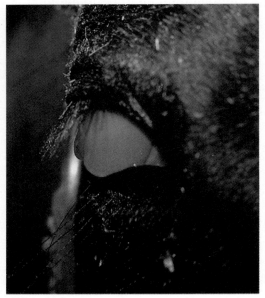

Edema of eye.

Corneal Ulcer with blood vessel in-growth.

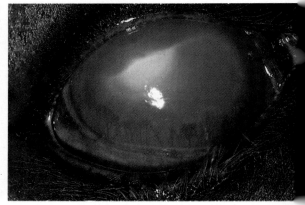

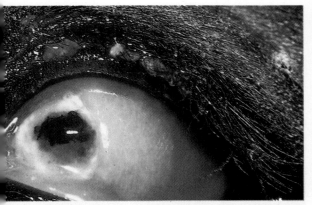

Full thickness corneal ulcer with trapped iris.

WHITE EYE OR WHITE SPOT ON EYE***

Possible Causes: Whitening of the cornea occurs with direct injury to the eye, or as a result of a systemic disease such as periodic ophthalmia (moon blindness).

Treatment: Same as for swollen eye. If available, instill antibiotic ointment or drops (no steroid added) every three to four hours, and atropine drops every four hours.

BLOOD IN EYE***

Possible Causes: May result from trauma or as a result of problem such as periodic ophthalmia.

Treatment: Same as for whitening of eye.

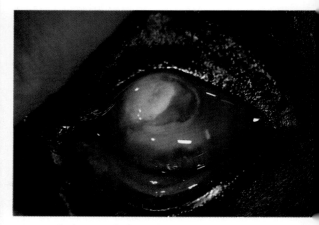

Corneal ulcer with fungal infection .

COLLAPSED EYE***

Cause: Penetrating injury, or erosion of an ulcer on the cornea.

Treatment: Same as for whitening of eye. If the eye is already under treatment (as for an ulcer), there must be a veterinary re-evaluation for any possible change in medications and injection of medications superficially into the sclera (white of the eye).

"BLOODSHOT" EYE

Possible Causes: Usually results from direct trauma to the eye. However, prominent blood vessels in the sclera may also be seen with other injuries or inflammations on the cornea or deep in the eye.

Treatment: There is no specific treatment for a "bloodshot" eye. This will resolve with treatment of other concurrent problems, as above.

PUS/WHITE MATERIAL AT CORNER OF EYE**

Possible Causes: Infection of any eye structures, inflammation of conjunctivae, blocked tear duct, or irritation from insects.

Treatment: Remove any accumulated material at frequent intervals with cool water. Apply fly repellants no closer than 1.4 inch around margins of eyes. May use antibiotic ophthalmic ointment or drops every four hours. A veterinary consultation is needed to rule out a blocked tear duct and to advise on use of medications containing steroids. Equine eyes are uniquely sensitive to steroids. Severe infection may follow their use if the cornea is even slightly injured.

SYMPTOM LIST

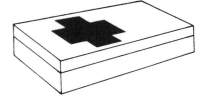

FIRST AID KIT

Blankets
Betadine solution
Zinc oxide or A & D skin ointments

CHAPTER XVIII

Frostbite and Exposure

DEFINITION:

Destruction of superficial tissues, with secondary damage to small blood vessels can result from exposure to severe cold. This is primarily a problem of foals, especially work foals, exposed to severe cold (windchill below 0° F). Other weakened animals are also at risk.

MILD FROSTBITE*

Signs include crusting of the muzzle and cold ear tips with initial loss of sensation.

Treatment: Hold a hot pack (105 to 108° F) to affected areas for 15 to 20 minutes. Then apply a mild antiseptic (e.g. Betadine solution), followed by ointment such as zinc oxide or A & D.

MODERATE FROSTBITE AND EXPOSURE**

Signs include the above plus a depressed body temperature (below 100° F for a foal, below 98° F for an older horse). Uncontrollable shivering may be present, with depression and sleepiness.

Treatment:
1. Treat superficially damaged areas as above.
2. Blanket and move the animal to a warmed area (a house in the case of a foal, a stall with heat lamps and/or a nearby space heater if the animal is larger), until temperature is normal.
3. Allow a foal free access to the mare and monitor the milk intake; call a veterinarian if the foal does not nurse in four hours.
4. Offer warm water and hot mash to an older horse.

SEVERE FROSTBITE AND EXPOSURE**

Signs include those for moderate frostbite and exposure, plus extremely cold feet. Feet that were kept under the body if the horse or foal was lying down will not be cold.

Treatment:
1. Treat as above for moderate exposure.
2. Stand a horse in buckets of warm water to encourage more rapid warming of the feet.
3. If a foal is lying down, wrap warm wet packs around the feet and change frequently.

COMPLICATIONS

Several days to weeks after the initial injury, dead tissues of the ears or feet, including hooves, may slough off.

Treatment:
1. Sloughing off of small areas at tips of ears should be treated as any open wound.
2. Animals which begin to show lameness and signs of oozing and separation at the coronary band may have to be put to sleep (euthanasia). Consult with your veterinarian as to the appropriate course of action.

SYMPTOM LIST

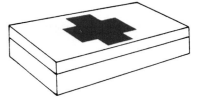

FIRST AID KIT

A & D ointment
Antibacterial wound cream
Antibiotic injection (if ordered by veterinarian)
Cold pack
Mild soap
Silver sulfadiazine cream
Sterile gauze pads
Zinc oxide

CHAPTER XIX

Lightning and Electric Shock

Injury or, more often, death results from contact with high electrical current in lightning or electrical line. Animals may be electrocuted either by direct contact with the lightning/current or by the spread of the charge. Current will travel along tree roots and may cause electrification of a shallow area of water at some distance from the actual source. Tile drains may also spread a charge. Soils vary in their conductivity, with loam being the most effective conductor, followed by sand, clay, marble, chalk and rocky soil.

Treatment
1. Most animals are killed. A sign of electrocution is a branching, tree-like pattern of singe marks along the legs and sometimes the body. The finding of partially chewed food in the mouth and absence of any abnormal postmortem conditions also point to a sudden death such as electrocution.
2. Animals that do not die may be unconscious for several minutes to hours. There is no specific treatment other than general support. The animal should be kept from extremes of heat or cold, in a well-bedded

stall, with fresh water and high quality hay. There may be neurological signs such as staggering, increased sensitivity to touch or sound, depression, which persists for several days to weeks.

3. Any burns should be treated as detailed in the chapter on burns.

CAUTION: DO NOT TOUCH THE HORSE IF ANIMAL IS STILL IN CONTACT WITH ELECTRICITY SOURCE.

SYMPTOM LIST

DISORDERS OF
URINE/URINATION

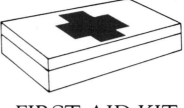

FIRST AID KIT

Liniment
Phenylbutazone
Thermometer

CHAPTER XX

Disorders of Urine/Urination

STRAINING TO URINATE* to**

Signs: Frequent stretching out as if to urinate (e.g. extending hind legs and dropping penis or opening lips of vulva) without passage of urine or with only a few drops of urine.

Causes:
1. Nonspecific abdominal pain.
2. Estrus (heat) in mares.
3. Stones in bladder or urethra (tube leading to outside from bladder).
4. Bladder infection.

What to Do: Try to rule out colic (see chapter on Disorders of Eating/Colic) and estrus behavior. Check stall to see if it is as wet as normal, i.e. if horse has been urinating. Observe horse carefully to see if he is able to urinate at all. If blockage is suspected, get immediate veterinary attention. DO NOT USE HOME REMEDIES OR OVER-THE-COUNTER REMEDIES FOR "KIDNEY PROBLEMS." These do not work and will cause delay in treatment of a blockage. If horse is urinating, try to catch a sample for analysis. (Moving the horse to a stall with clean bedding often triggers urination.)

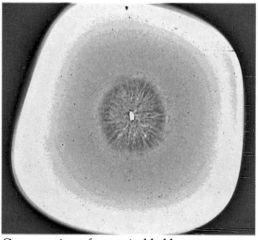

Cross section of stone in bladder

FREQUENT URINATION* to**

Signs: Same as above, with passage of small amount of urine each time.

Causes: Same as above.

What to Do: Same as above.

DISCOLORED URINE* to**

Definition: Passage of urine which is any color other than yellow or whitish.

Causes: Normal horse urine is yellow to whitish, the white color being due to the large amount of crystals normally present. Urine may be very dark if it is highly concentrated, as will be the first urine of the morning or if water intake has not been adequate. Dark urine may also occur with destruction of red blood cells (red cell pigment), liver disease (bile pigment), or muscle breakdown (muscle pigment). Red urine may also be seen with bladder infections or stones, or with tumors of the urinary tract (rare).

What to Do: Take horse's temperature (may be elevated with an infection). Observe for signs of colic from urinary tract pain. Obtain a sample of urine for the veterinarian to analyse. (You can bring this to the office and both save a farm call and have the veterinarian prepared for any necessary further work-up when he does come out.)

"SORE KIDNEYS"

Definition: "Sore kidneys" is a term horsemen often use to refer to tenderness along the topline of the back, in the general area of the saddle.

Causes: In fact, kidney soreness that you can detect by pressure along the back is rarely, if ever, present. Tenderness in this area is caused by back strain, either from pulling a load, lameness in the hindlegs causing the horse to move stiffly and abnormally, or primary back muscle stiffness due to underlying spinal problems. If any other signs of urinary problems are present (see above)—and they surely would be if there were kidney pain— obtain a urine sample for analysis. For muscular back pain, rest the horse for three days, massage back with strong liniment after applying moist hot towels three times a day, keep the horse blanketed in cool weather, and give phenylbutazone, two grams once daily. If no improvement after three days, get veterinary evaluation.

SYMPTOM LIST

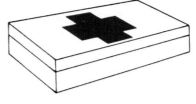

FIRST AID KIT

Banamine
Phenylbutazone
Antibiotic ointment
Sling for penis

CHAPTER XXI

Reproductive Organs

DROPPED PENIS

Definition: The correct term for a persistently dropped penis is paraphimosis (a temporary condition often) or priapism (a paralysed penis).

Causes of Paraphimosis: Equine infectious Anemia (EIA), purpura hemorrhagica (blood poisoning), rhinopneumonitis, exhaustion, starvation, or paralysed penis, trauma or infection of penis/sheath or drug reaction (phenothiazine tranquilizers).

Treatment of Paraphimosis: With trauma or infection of the penis or sheath, the area should be cleansed well and cold water hosing performed for 15 to 20 minutes four times daily to minimize edema. With infection or direct injury to the penis, the penis should be coated with an antibiotic ointment and antibiotic injections may be indicated. Anti-inflammatory therapy with phenylbutazone or Banamine is indicated for three to five days. Supporting the penis in a sling—either a specifically manufactured stallion support or a sheet tied around the belly—may be needed. Get veterinary advice regarding treatment if not resolved in 3 days. With paraphimosis of other causes, support and time are the only treatments.

Causes of Priapism: Injury to local nerves, rabies, phenothiazine tranquilizers.

Treatment of Priapism: True penile paralysis is treated by amputation of the penis, after the stage of acute inflammation caused by blood pooling has subsided. In the interim, penile support is indicated.

TRAUMA TO PENIS

See paraphimosis, above.

SWELLING OF SHEATH (PREPUCE)

Causes: May be caused by injury (see paraphimosis, above) or by collection of secretions in the sheath and secondary skin irritation and

Prepucial edema .

infection. The surface of the extended penis will be covered with flaky and/or dark tarry material.

Treatment: See paraphimosis, above.

TRAUMA TO VULVA

Causes: Trauma to the vulva can occur during breeding, foaling (see appropriate chapter), abuse by caretakers or accidental injury.

Treatment: Cleanse area with gentle soap and hose with cold water 3 times daily for 15 to 20 minutes. Extensive tears will require suturing. Superficial lacerations should be covered with an antibiotic ointment.

COLIC FOLLOWING BREEDING***

Cause: Perforation of vagina by penis.

Treatment: Any colic occurring within 24 hours of breeding could be from perforation of the vagina and is a medical emergency. The penis will carry contamination directly into the abdominal cavity and an extensive and life-threatening infection results. Do not attempt to treat this on your own.

SYMPTOM LIST

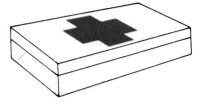

FIRST AID KIT

Large amount sterile lubricant such as K-Y Jelly

Equipment to apply traction on foal if needed—obstetrical chains or substitute such as lightweight chains (e.g. dog choke collars) or belts (leather or nylon)

Several heavy towels

Blanket

Acepromazine or Rompun tranquilizer

Banamine for pain relief

Dipyrone or Jenotone for colic pain

Rubber gloves with textured fingers

CHAPTER XXII

Foaling

PROLONGED LABOR/FAILURE OF FOAL TO APPEAR ** to ***

Definition: Active labor with active straining for longer than 20 to 25 minutes.

What to Do: Allow mare to roll if she wants to. This is a natural response and helps to reposition a foal that is not properly aligned in the birth canal. Check the vagina to make sure it has not been partially sewn shut (Caslick's operation—a common procedure to help prevent infections). If she is sewn up, you will have to open this along the scar by inserting one clean hand in the vagina and spreading the fingers just behind the vaginal opening to stretch the tissues tight. The center of the sutured area will be evident as a thin, white scar. This area has no sensation and can be cut with a scissors. If previous Caslick's surgery is not the problem, wash hands and arms well with soap and water but leave them wet. Insert a hand in the vagina and feel around for the foal's feet or nose or any part of the foal. Foals are rarely too large to fit through the birth canal, as long as they are positioned properly. If you can feel part of the foal in the vagina, push it back as far as possible during a rest period between contractions and straining. Then allow the mare to move around and roll.

When to call the veterinarian: With this, or any problem with foaling, call the veterinarian as soon as you suspect a problem. It is also a good idea to locate any local horsemen experienced in foaling who might be available to help on short notice.

IMPROPER POSITIONING OF FOAL **to ***

Most foals are born with the nose resting on the front legs and one foot slightly further forward than the other. However, they can also be born hind legs first without a problem. When the feet first appear, it may look as if the foal is lying on his side or even upside down. However, this too will correct itself as the foal moves further along. If only one foot is present, the leg may be hung up at the elbow (or hock). To correct this, the foal must be pushed back, as described above, and the trapped leg then grasped above the foot and pulled forward. Wrap the mare's tail and wash the genital area with mild soap, then rinse with water. Wash your hands and arms and apply K-Y Jelly, clean Vaseline or other lubricant (an appropriate lubricant should always be part of your foaling kit). This is best done by looping a light weight chain (such as a dog choke collar) or a belt either above or below the trapped fetlock and pulling out and down toward the mare's hocks. Again, intervention by experienced personnel is preferred but you cannot afford to wait too long if the foal is already partially along the birth canal, as the umbilical cord is being compressed.

FAILURE OF FOAL TO ADVANCE** to***

Occasionally, part of the foal will be visible but delivery becomes arrested. If the problem is a simple elbow or hock hang-up (see above), proceed as already described. If only one foot is present, you will have to locate the other foot and bring it forward. To do this, push the foal back as far as possible, between contractions. Follow the leg that is present up to the body. Keeping your hand on the chest (or hind-quarters), travel to the other side and locate the other leg. Follow this leg down to the foot, cup the foot in the palm of your hand and rotate it away from the foal's body and toward the flank of the mare while pushing back on the body with the other hand. Then carefully pull the foot and leg back toward you until the leg is straightened out. Delivery can then proceed normally. The above described maneuver is difficult to perform and will seem to take forever. However, if you remain calm and proceed slowly and cautiously, the chance of success is good. If you are unable to accomplish this, keep pushing the foal back as far as possible until help arrives. Occasionally, the foal will become trapped at the shoulders. If this happens, the foal will have the neck and most of the front legs out. To correct this, push the foal back several inches, then grasp one foot and pull it forward further than the other. This will allow one shoulder at a time to enter the pelvis. Once positioned, grasp the legs and gently pull down toward the hocks as the mare strains to deliver the foal. Follow the same procedure if the foal is presenting hind legs first and is hung up at the pelvis.

UTERINE EXHAUSTION
(ATONY)**

With prolonged and difficult labors, the uterus may cease to contract and the mare's urge to push is lost. If the foal is not positioned correctly, this condition actually benefits the person trying to manipulate the foal, as there will be no resistance. Regardless of how the foal is positioned, it will have to be delivered by the birth attendant. Grasp the two front feet of the foal, keeping one leg slightly behind the other, and exert gentle, steady traction backwards and down on an angle parallel with the hocks. If the mare is standing (and they often are with a hard labor), someone should be positioned to break the foal's fall and prevent sudden rupture of the cord. If the foal is slippery, use the traction devices mentioned above or try a pair of rubber kitchen/utility gloves with textured fingers to get a better grip. Do not cut the cord; allow it to break naturally in the course of the foal moving around. Then tie it off (if bleeding) about two inches from the belly with heavy cord or baling twine. DO NOT pull on the placenta to remove it. This can cause it to break.

PREMATURE RUPTURE OF
CORD **

The umbilical cord will break on its own as the mare and foal move around. If ruptured too early, heavy bleeding could occur—blood that should have gone into the foal. The foal may then be weak, short of breath and have difficulty standing and nursing (see below). If foal has not made substantial efforts to stand in two

hours and nurse in three hours, get emergency
veterinary attention.

WEAK MARE POSTPARTUM ***

The mare is normally quite tired after foaling and will remain lying down for around 20
minutes or so. This is beneficial, as it allows all
the blood from the placenta time to enter the
foal before movement of dam and foal causes
the cord to break. However, internal injuries
or hemorrhage may be what is keeping the
mare down.

What to Do: Take the mare's pulse, temperature and respiration. These should be in the
normal range in about 20 minutes after foaling.
Check the color of the mucous membranes of
her mouth. If very pale, suspect hemorrhage.
Observe the mare's general attitude. Even if
still down, she should be alert and looking
back at the foal, calling the foal or nuzzling it.
If she is depressed, anxious or oblivious to the
foal, this is abnormal. Relay the above information to the veterinarian. Dry the foal with a
thick towel if drying has not been done by the
mare. Place the foal close to her body, preferably where it can nurse when lying down, and
blanket the mare.

COLIC IN MARE POSTPARTUM ***

Signs of colic in the mare or contractions of
the uterus suggest possible injury to abdominal
organs or hemorrhage. (See above for what to do
if mare is down.) If mare is up and agitated, care
must be taken that she does not injure the foal.
Dipyrone (10 mg./lb.), Jenotone (0.25mg./lb.),

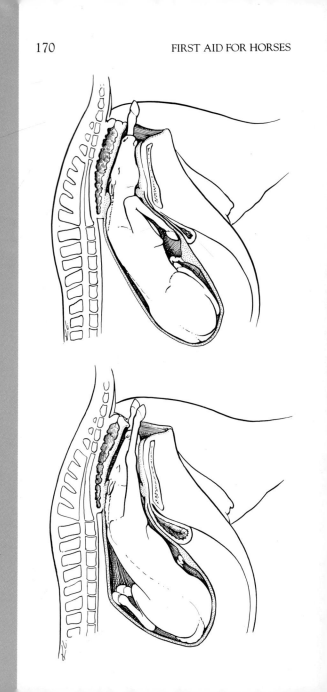

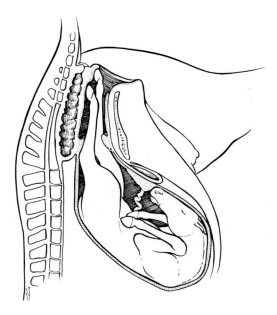

Above-

A hindfeet first presentation of a foal.

Top, left-

A foal, with one front leg in a normal presentation
and the other flexed back under the body, with
chest/shoulder area pressed against the brim of the
pelvis, and normally positioned foot in birth canal.

Bottom, left-

A foal in normal position, with feet in vagina
during labor.

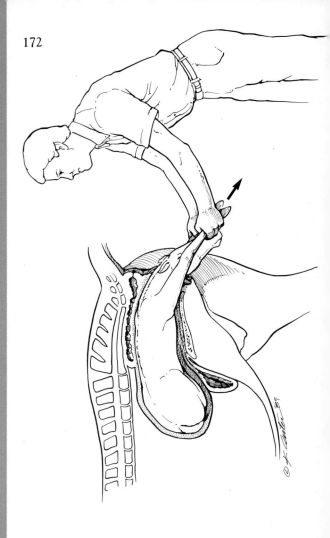

or Banamine (0.5mg./lb.) may be tried to control any pain, but tranquilizers should be avoided. If mare becomes violent, remove the foal to outside the doorway to the stall, but leave door open. Have someone hold the foal and another person remain at the doorway to control the mare, if necessary. This arrangement protects the foal but limits separation anxiety.

REJECTION OF FOAL**

Some mares will reject their foals for reasons that are unclear. This is more common with maiden mares, but may happen at any time, with any mare. The mare may refuse to have anything to do with the foal or may only resist having it nurse. Try having someone hold up one of the mare's front legs while you milk out some colostrum and then allow the foal to nurse when she has accepted this. If still actively resistant, a low dose of tranquilizer may be all that is needed to overcome anxiety and allow the mare and foal to bond. If this is given within two to three hours of birth, the udder will still be full and minimal amounts will reach the foal. Use 10 to 20 mg. of Acepromazine or 100 mg. of Rompun intramuscularly. Once this has taken effect, someone should stand at the mare's head while another person helps the foal to nurse. If this barrier can be overcome, the mare will sometimes grant a grudging acceptance of the foal that at least is sufficient for the foal to survive. If she is still actively resistant, seek professional advice immediately.

SYMPTOM LIST

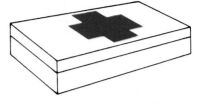

FIRST AID KIT

Enemas
Glycerin suppositories
Thermometer

CHAPTER XXIII

Newborn Emergencies

The normal newborn foal is lively, alert and very active. Although his initial attempts to stand are very wobbly and uncoordinated, he makes repeated and energetic tries. The first 6 to 12 hours after birth are critical. The foal must receive the mare's first milk (colostrum) well within this time frame, and in adequate amounts to obtain the rich supply of antibodies it contains. The foal's energy, electrolyte and fluid stores are also low, and intake of the mare's milk is essential to life. If you even suspect the foal is not normal, it is best to get immediate veterinary attention so that steps can be taken to get that all-important first milk into the foal and to evaluate the baby to try to uncover and correct the problem.

FAILURE TO STAND ***

The foal's first attempts to stand usually occur within 30 to 60 minutes after birth. He may begin by hopping around like a gigantic frog, but eventually gets several legs, then all four, under him. Stance at first is wide-based (splayed out) but comes to resemble normal as strength and confidence are gained.

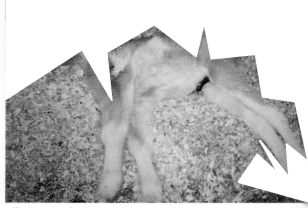

Prostrate foal .

When to Get Help: The time span from birth to standing is highly variable. However, if by two hours the foal has not managed to stand, but otherwise appears normal, you can assist him to his feet and help to steady him. Once this barrier is past, a normal foal will quickly become more proficient and able to accomplish this on his own.

If the foal is weak, disinterested or seems depressed, place several fingers in his mouth. If a good, strong sucking reflex is present, he may be able to nurse if you hold him up to the mare's udder. Once he has nursed (note for how long and at what age, in hours, this occurred), seek veterinary attention if he is not significantly stronger after 20 to 30 minutes. If the foal was not able to nurse well, you will need veterinary assistance to pass a stomach tube to feed the foal.

FAILURE TO NURSE***

If the foal has successfully gained his feet but has not nursed, or attempted to nurse, in 2 to 3 hours, guide him back to the udder and express a little milk onto your fingers. Once the foal is sucking the fingers, bring them close to the udder, extricate your fingers and gently guide the nipple into his mouth. (This sounds easier than it is; be patient.) Once a normal foal has successfully nursed, he is unlikely to have further problems.

If the foal is up and moving but seems abnormal in any way—wandering around, bumping into things, making abnormal sounds —and cannot be guided to nurse, as described above, get immediate veterinary attention.

FAILURE TO PASS MANURE**

The fecal material present in the foal's gastrointestinal tract at birth is a sticky, dark, pasty manure. Constipation in new foals is a fairly common problem (some breeding operations even routinely give enemas to newborns to prevent this) and may be more common in colts than fillies. The foal should be carefully observed in the first 12 to 24 hours to guarantee it is passing manure frequently and that the manure is not overly dry. Wholly or partially constipated foals will strain often without result. The problem can become quite serious if not corrected early.

What to Do: If the foal shows the above signs of impaction, you can give him an enema, using a commercial preparation such as

Fleet's enema (available in drug stores). If the enema meets with minimal or little success, insert several glycerin suppositories into the anus. Wait an hour, and if the foal is still straining unsuccessfully, the enema may be repeated. If this is still not successful, the veterinarian should be brought in.

FAILURE TO URINATE***

The foal should also be observed carefully to see that it is urinating normally. Rupture of the bladder can occur during birth. This will result in colic and depression within 24 hours of birth. Prior to that, no urination or passage of only small amounts of urine will be noted. If urination is suspected to be abnormal, get immediate veterinary attention.

Abdominal pain, foal .

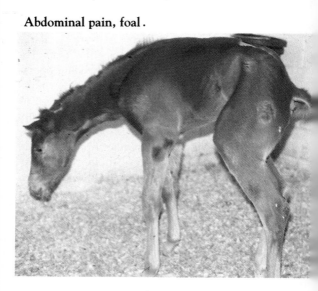

Small amounts of urine may also be noted when the urachus, a connection between the bladder and placenta in the fetus, does not close over normally. In these foals, urine may be seen coming from the umbilical cord area. This can often be taken care of with simple procedures, but does require veterinary attention.

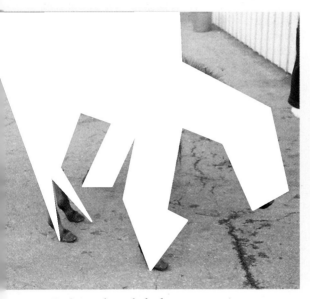

Deformed weak foal.

WEAK OR DEPRESSED FOALS***

As mentioned above, the normal newborn foal is extremely lively and alert, attentive to all things around him. His movements are strong, if not always coordinated. Any deviation from this is cause for concern. The problem may be as simple as a low blood sugar or a complicated neurological condition. In any case, foals that remain depressed and weak for longer than 20 to 30 minutes after birth should immediately be evaluated for special care.

HYPOTHERMIA **

While even very young foals can survive birth in cold conditions, extremely frigid weather, particularly if combined with a difficult birth, can overcome his capacities and dangerous hypothermia (subnormal temperature) sets in. The foal's energy stores can be rapidly used up in trying to generate enough body heat. Any foal with a body temperature below 98° should be warmed with active rubbing, heat lamps or even removal to a heated area until he returns to normal temperature.

COMMON DRUG REACTIONS

CHAPTER XXIV

Some Common Drug Reactions

This chapter by no means covers all the possible drug reactions. Some are mild and not true emergencies, and therefore not mentioned. Others are only applicable to drugs that should be administered only by a veterinarian, and are acute reactions which would occur while the veterinarian was still present. The drug reactions chosen for inclusion refer to agents that are commonly administered by the horse owner or trainer or are reactions that could occur after the veterinarian has given a drug and left the farm.

ANTIBIOTICS

Procaine penicillin

Some horses develop an "allergy" to procaine penicillin (the intramuscular form of penicillin) characterized by twitching, agitation and excitability within 5 to 15 minutes of administration. It is unclear whether this is a true penicillin allergy or a reaction to the procaine or to too rapid absorption of the drug secondary to direct injection into a vessel, or to injection into a muscular site previously used for multiple injections where tissue damage resulted in a greater than normal blood supply. In any case, there is no specific treatment called for and the reaction will pass on its own. However, that horse should not receive any further procaine penicillin.

Tetracycline

Tetracycline is given intravenously by the veterinarian, usually to treat a lung infection. Horses carrying a salmonella infection may develop a full-blown case of salmonella diarrhea during the course of treatment with tetracycline. If diarrhea of any degree develops, isolate the horse and alert the veterinarian.

Sulfa drugs

Although rare, horses with low-level renal function problems may have trouble handling sulfa drugs and develop renal failure. This should be considered if a horse on sulfas develops depression or decreased appetite or generally seems ill for no apparent reason.

-mycin drugs (Gentamicin, Streptomycin, etc.)

These can cause renal failure in high doses or when given to very ill animals. See sulfa antibiotics, above.

TRANQUILIZERS

Accidental injection of tranquilizers into an artery, instead of a vein, can cause severe reactions. The promazine group given intra-arterially may cause profound sedation and a rapid drop in blood pressure, even collapse. When xylazine (Rompun) is given into an artery, extreme agitation occurs. To avoid this, intravenous injections should be given as low down in the neck as possible, as the vein and artery are close together in the upper neck. Better yet, injections given without a veterinarian present to give emergency treatment should be given intramuscularly. In the event of collapse (with this or any other drug), give epinephine, 1:1000 strength, 4 to 8 cc, in muscle or under the skin. FOLLOW DIRECTIONS ON BOTTLE. Carefully read them in advance of any such emergency.

WORMERS

All worming preparations are capable of causing the horse to go off feed, even show mild signs of colic. This should resolve in a day or so, but it is wise to withhold grain in horses reacting poorly, and to check the feet routinely for signs of laminitis. Laminitis was more of a problem with the older preparations for bots that had to be administered by stomach tube than with today's paste formulas.

Another precaution is to avoid giving phenothiazine tranquilizers to horses that have received a worming preparation containing Dyrex in the previous days, as the effect of the tranquilizer may be magnified.

B VITAMINS

Injectable B vitamins are commonly used by trainers, either alone or in combination with intravenous fluids, to combat stress during periods of heavy competition. However, there is a fairly high incidence of adverse reactions, ranging from trembling and weakness to collapse and even death. Reactions can occur even in a horse that has previously received injectable B vitamins without any problems. High doses given rapidly are most likely to cause the problem, but there is no 100-percent safe way to inject B vitamins in horses. Giving a test dose of approximately ⅓ the total dose by the intramuscular route and observing the horse for 15 minutes will pick up some of the horses that are hypersensitive, but is no guarantee against reactions. The best solution is not to give them at all, or to have the veterinarian do it. In event of collapse, use epinephine (see Tranquilizers, above).

Even oral B vitamin supplementation may cause problems. Large doses of thiamine can cause tranquilization. Niacin or even multiple B supplements in large doses can cause excitement.

REACTIONS AT INTRAMUSCULAR INJECTION SITES

All drugs and vaccines given intramuscularly carry the risk of tissue reaction ranging from heat, swelling and pain to actual abscess formation. This is most likely to occur with some vaccinations (e.g. flu or "Strangles") and with any drug where the label clearly states to give by deep intramuscular injection only. Intramuscular injection of a drug intended only for intravenous use (e.g. phenylbutazone) is almost guaranteed to produce tissue damage. These reactions, even an abscess, are not emergencies, although veterinary attention may be needed to open, drain and flush the area. However, if the tissue becomes blackened or develops a peculiar crackling texture when you run your hand over the skin (meaning there is gas in the tissues), immediate veterinary attention is needed. This latter reaction signifies the presence of a gas-producing bacterium, which could be fatal.

PHENYLBUTAZONE AND OTHER ANTI-INFLAMMATORY DRUGS

These agents are capable of causing irritation—even ulceration—of the gastrointestinal tract which in turn results in decreased appetite, particularly for grain, and even signs of mild colic. Individual increased sensitivity or an underlying irritation (e.g. bots in the stomach) may result in problems a short time after starting treatment. Generally, however,

Injection abcess of hindquarters, left.

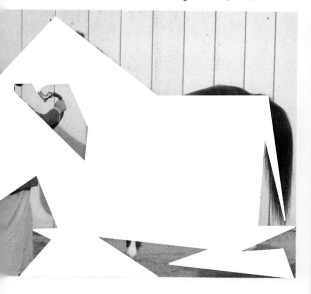

this is a complication of long-term and/or high-dose therapy. You can try giving the drug only after the horse has eaten, mixing it in 30cc of Milk of Magnesia to make a slurry to deliver by oral syringe. If this does not alleviate symptoms, discontinue the drug.

Important Emergency Information for the Veterinarian

Age, breed, sex and use of the horse.

Temperature, pulse and respiratory rate (TPR) (*See Appendix 7*)

Appetite and water consumption.

Amount and any changes in manure.

Nature of problem, if known
- symptoms?

Has horse ever had this problem before
- when
- diagnosis then
- treatments
- response to treatments?

When did symptoms start
- have they worsened, improved or remained the same?

If bleeding, how much?

Has horse received any treatment yet?

Is the horse on any medications regularly or been treated with any drugs recently (including wormers, tranquilizers, etc.)

Is the horse allergic or unusually sensitive to any medication?

APPENDIX 2

Emergency Phone Numbers

Regular Veterinarian ________________________

____

Back up Veterinarians ______________________

____

____

Full Service Veterinary Hospital ______________

____

Agricultural Extension Agent _________________

Poison Control Center ______________________

Rescue Squad __________________________

Vanning _______________________________

Fire Company/Fire Rescue __________________

Police: Local ____________________________

State ____________________________

Insurance Company ________________________

____

____

General Signs of Serious Illness

1. Refusal to eat or drink/inability to eat or drink
2. Watery diarrhea/constipation
3. Inability to walk or stand
4. Fever over 101°
5. Labored or noisy breathing/rapid breathing
6. Pulse greater than 80
7. Dramatic change in behavior (either depression or agitation)
8. Straining to urinate or red/brown urine
9. Bleeding for any reason that does not stop in 5 to 10 minutes or bright red bleeding that pulsates
10. Severe edema (swelling) of legs and/or along lower abdomen
11. Seizure

Signs of Adequate Tranquilization

1. Head held low
2. Drooping eyelids
3. Drooping lower lip, ears
4. Penis relaxed
5. Wide-based stance in front
6. Noisy breathing*

*Not a necessary sign—indicates moderate to heavy tranquilization with partial paralysis of the throat. Remove hay, feed and water until breathing returns to normal.

NOTE: The horse must be observed from a distance. Any horse may be temporarily aroused to a state of alertness when handled. The horse can still kick, strike, etc. when tranquilized. However, his reactions will be much slower and it will usually take more stimulus to cause the undesired reaction.

Shock membranes.

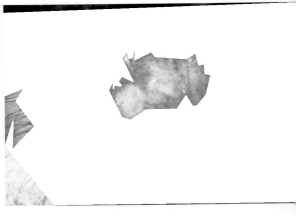

Signs of Shock

1. Weakness
2. Trembling
3. Depression
4. Cold ears
5. Cold extremities
6. Rapid, weak pulse
7. Pale mucous membranes
8. Decreased capillary refill time
9. Decreased urinary output

Bandaging

ROUTINE STANDING LEG WRAP

Place quilted cotton wrap such that the beginning and end lie across the front of the cannon bone, not on the tendons. To begin the outer, elastic wrap, tuck the end under the edge of the finished cotton wrap (Photo VI-A) ½ to ⅓ of the way up the leg. Angle the wrap downward and carefully encircle the leg, keeping the pressure even and avoiding all wrinkles (Photo VI-B). Overlap the layer above (or below as you work back up) for a width of ⅓ to ½ the width of the wrap (Photo VI-C). If desired, at the back of the ankle (fetlock) you can make one or two loops that travel under the sesamoids and back of the joint, to provide extra support and relief from strain (Photo VI-D). Finally, change directions smoothly, avoiding wrinkles, and work back up the leg to finish the wrap at the top of the leg (Photo VI-E).

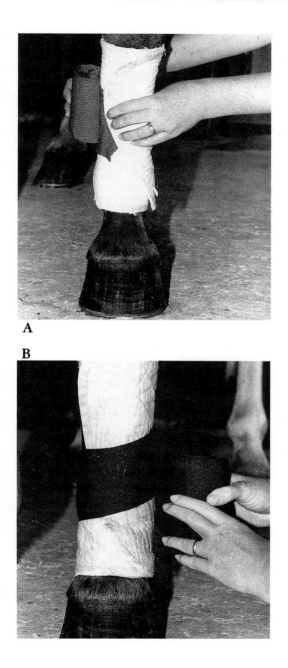

A

B

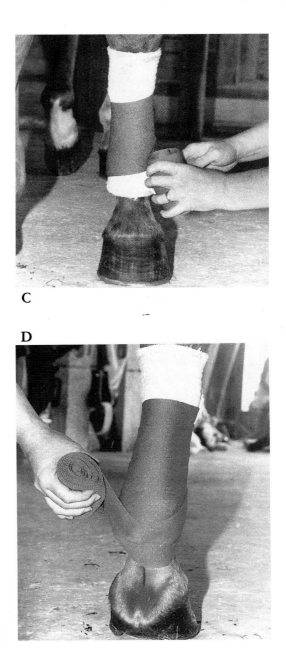

C

D

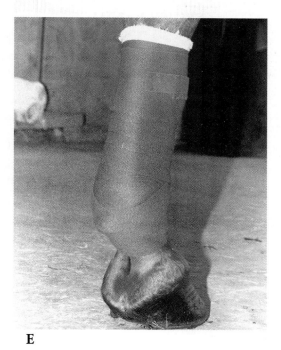

E

SPIDER BANDAGE

Spider bandages are used to apply pressure to the knee joint area. They are designed not to slip down when the horse moves his leg. To make a spider, cut a sufficient length of muslin to span six to eight inches above and below the knee. Fold the material in half and, using scissors, cut strips into the material ¾ to 1 inch wide (Photo VI-F). These will be braided down the outside of the leg with the uncut portion resting on the inside and front of the leg (VI-G). To begin, tie a knot with the first two strips. (VI-H). Then, progress down the leg, braiding tightly. As your middle strand becomes too short, use the finished braid above for a new middle strand (VI-H). When finished, tuck the bottom edges neatly underneath (VI-I). Spiders may also be applied over standing bandages or over dressings, ice packs, etc. on the knee itself.

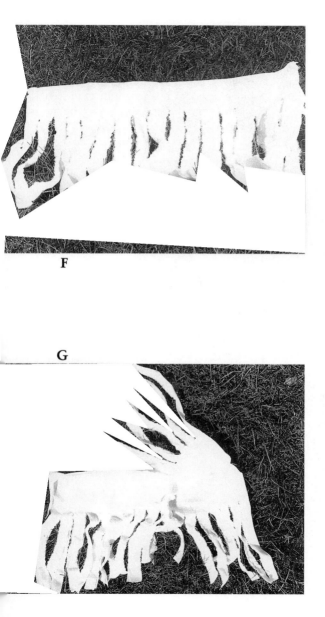

F

G

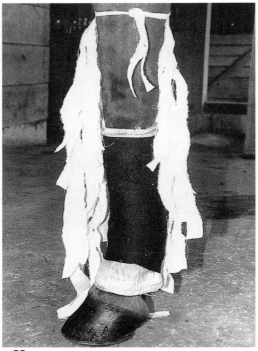

H

I

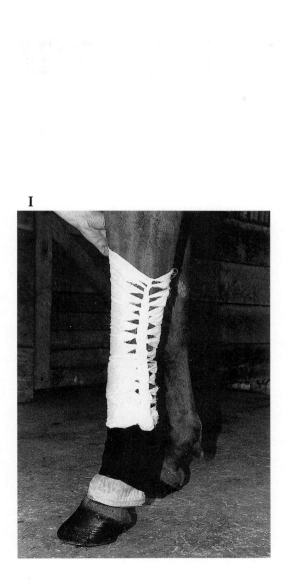

FIGURE OF EIGHT WRAP

The figure of eight wrap is another way to apply pressure across the knee and is also useful for the hock. Begin the wrap by encircling the leg once or twice below the hock (or knee) (Photo VI-J). Next, angle the wrap up across the front of the joint, from inside to outside (VI-K). Next, make two loops above the joint, then begin downward again, crossing the joint from inside to outside to make an "X" (Photo VI-L). Repeat the crisscrossing several times, making loops above and below the joint as well as needed to stabilize the wrap and keep it from slipping down. Finish the wrap, either above or below the joint, with a straight encircling loop. Note that when doing the hock, the point of the hock is left free to allow the leg to move. Similarly, when doing a knee, the prominent accessory carpal bone at the back of the knee is left free. (Figure VI-M)

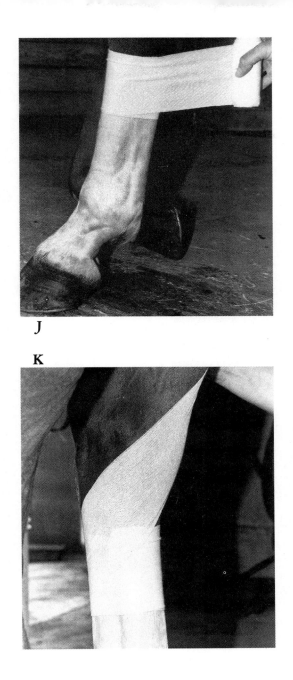

J

K

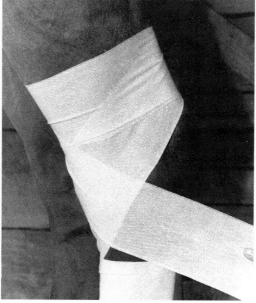

L

M

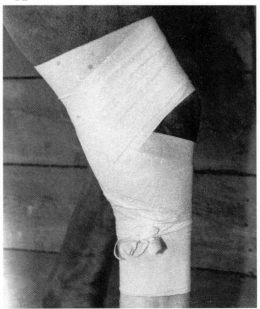

Recording Temperature, Pulse and Respiration

The horse's temperature, pulse and respiration are termed his "vital signs," since they reflect the general health of some of his vital systems (heart, lungs, immune system, temperature regulation) and also, nonspecifically, show whether the horse is distressed in any way. They are also important barometers of how a problem is progressing—becoming more abnormal if the condition worsens and returning toward normal as the horse improves. Whenever you suspect a problem, recording the horse's temperature, pulse and respiration (TPR) should be among the first steps you take.

Temperature (Photo VII-A)

The horse's temperature is taken rectally, using a special horse thermometer which is larger and stronger than the human counterpart. To prevent losing the thermometer into the rectum, attach a string to the hole located at the end of the thermometer and from there to a clothes pin or other suitable clip. The thermometer assembly may then be safely clipped to the tail hairs. Cool water, vaseline or other gel lubricant may be used to ease insertion. Stand to the side of the horse, not directly behind, and close to his body. Move the tail to the side to visualize the anus and insert the thermometer. This should be left in for approximately 2 minutes for an accurate reading (try to avoid inserting it into fecal material which will give false readings). Normal values are anywhere between 98° and 100° (rarely as high as 100.5 or 101°) for an adult horse at rest, depending on individual variation and the weather conditions.

A

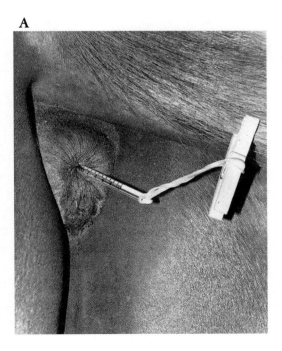

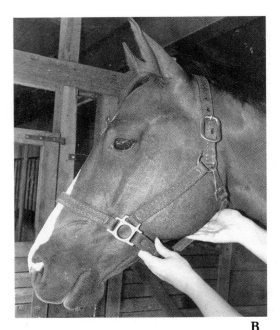

B

Pulse

The pulse is taken by gently pressing the fingertips against an artery that is close to the surface of the skin. The best location for this is along the curve of the cheek muscle. The blood vessels there can be easily felt and rolling under the skin. Wait until you can feel the pulse clearly and then count the number of beats per minute (or beats per 15 seconds and multiply by four). Normal pulse is anywhere from the high 20s to the low 40s, depending on how excited the horse is at the time, as well as on his level of fitness and the weather.

Respiration

The respiratory rate is taken by observing the movement of the ribs (out as he inhales, in as he exhales) and counting the number of breaths per minute, as described above for pulse. Normal respiratory rate is approximately 8 to 16 breaths per minute, with the rate being influenced by the same factors as described above for temperature and pulse.

Twitching the Horse

Although it seems unusually cruel to some people, twitching is a basic and often quite necessary method of restraint, particularly when dealing with an injured and/or frightened horse.

While it would seem that twitches of any sort should cause pain, it has been shown that the horse's respiratory and heart rates actually fall when he is twitched, much as if under the effect of a tranquilizer, and not at all as would be expected if the horse was in considerable pain.

To place the twitch, stand with one hand on the halter and the other, with the loop of the twitch resting on the handler's wrist, grasping the nose. (Photo VIII-A). Grab hold of a generous portion of the nose and slip the loop of the twitch over the hand and onto the nose. The other hand then leaves the halter and turns the twitch to tighten the loop around the nose (Photo VIII-B). Alternately, a second person can tighten the twitch. Once tight, apply sufficient constant twist to the handle to prevent it from loosening and falling off—the amount of pressure needed to be decided by how much resistance the horse is giving. (Photo VIII-C).

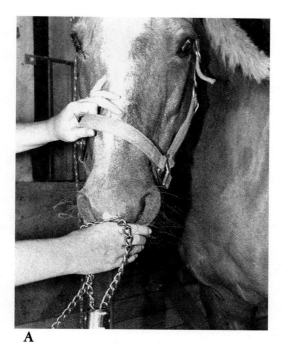

A

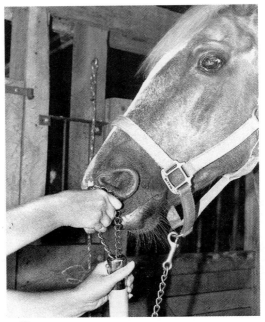

B

C

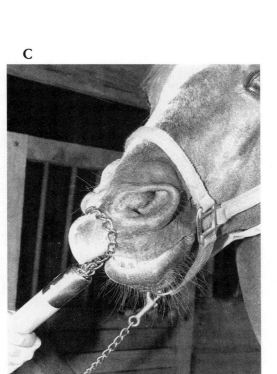

APPENDIX 9

Giving Intramuscular Injections

Begin by identifying the proper anatomical area. This photo shows the safe area for the most popular injection site, the neck. Prepare the site by brushing off loose dirt and hair, washing with soap and water and wiping (down to skin level) with alcohol. **A**

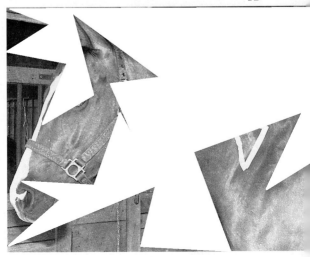

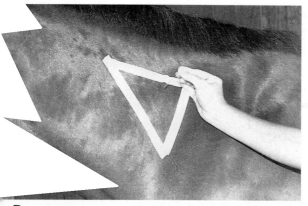

B   Hold the needle between thumb and first finger, touching only the hub (top). Aim for the center of your target area and *quickly and forcefully* place the needle deep into the muscle. This should be done in a manner very similar to shooting a dart. Slow insertion, or hesitant insertion, causes much more pain. Also, do not slap or punch the horse before inserting needle. This does *not* numb the area but does make the horse upset.

This needle is properly inserted, straight into the muscle for its full length.

C

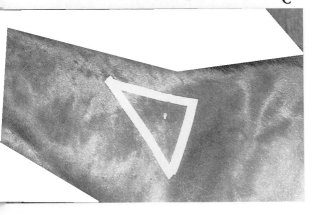

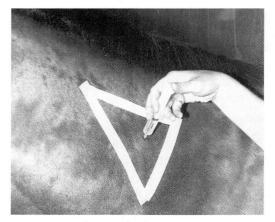

Next, securely attach the syringe containing the medication and inject at a slow and steady pace.

Since necks often become sore after multiple injections, alternate sites are needed. The best is the large muscle mass of the upper hind leg.

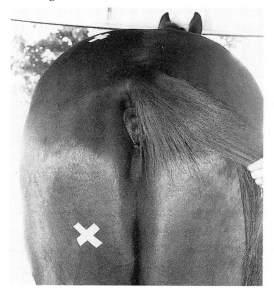

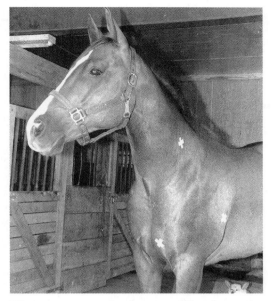

There are several other possible alternative sites which may be used. However, always clear use of these sites with your veterinarian first.

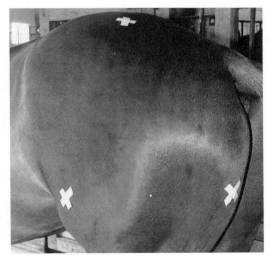

Administering Eye Medications

Eye medications can be easily given after a little practice. However, it is always best to have a helper since you will need both hands free.

The eye is first held open by pressing on the skin above and under the limits of the eyeball with the thumb and first or second finger, pulling upward on the upper eyelid and down on the lower eyelid (photo X-A).

Steady the hand holding the medication by resting it firmly against the horse's head. Position the tube or bottle of medication at about a 45-degree angle to the eye and ¼ to ½ inch above the level of the eye. Hold this position fixed and follow the movements of the horse's head at all times to avoid directly contacting and/or possibly injuring the eye. Place medication directly onto the surface of the eye, then allow eyelids to close. (Photo X-B).

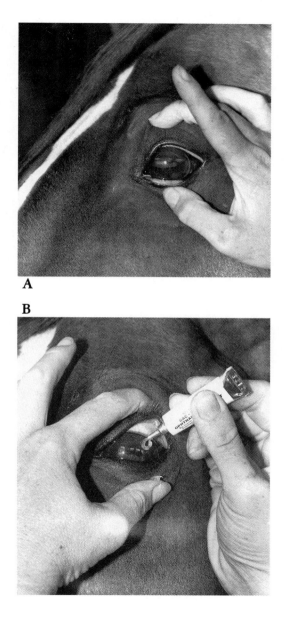

A

B

Glossary of some Possibly Unfamiliar Terms

Abscess: A pocket of infection located deeply in the muscles or elsewhere in the body, surrounded by a thick wall of tissue.

Analgesic: Substance which controls pain.

Antihistamine: Class of drug which blocks allergic reactions.

Antibody: A protein produced by the immune system cells that attacks an infectious organism or other foreign substance in the body.

Antitoxin: An antibody against a toxin/poison produced by a bacterium.

Botulism: A type of food poisoning produced by the toxins secreted by the bacterium Clostridium botulinum, which causes progressive paralysis and usually death.

Caslick's Surgery: A very common surgery performed on mares, which sutures the lips of the vagina partially closed to prevent urine, manure or air entry.

Colic: Pain in the abdomen.

Contaminate: To allow infectious agents or foreign material (e.g. dirt) to enter the body —e.g. through a wound.

Cornea: The outer layer of the eye.

Dermatitis: Inflammation of the skin.

Dermatophilus: An organism that commonly infects the skin.

Edema: Swelling caused by accumulation of fluid in an inflamed area, by heart or kidney failure or following damage to the veins, arteries or lymphatic drainage system of an area.

Electrolyte: Salt that is normally present in the body and/or fed or injected to replace salts lost (e.g. sodium, potassium, chloride, bicarbonate).

Emphysema: Disease of lungs characterized by inability to completely empty out the air when breathing out.

Encephalomyelitis: Inflammation of brain and spinal cord.

Euthanasia: Humane destruction of the horse ("putting to sleep").

Expiration: Breathing out.

Founder: Laminitis, inflammation of the sensitive/live tissues of the hoof.

Foreign: Not normally found in the body.

Hyperthermia: Temperature above normal-fever.

Hypothermia: Temperature below normal.

Inspiration: Breathing in.

Intramuscular: Into a muscle.

Intravenous: Into a vein.

Jaundice: Yellow discoloration of the skin and mucus membranes (e.g. lining of the mouth) by pigments which accumulate in the body during liver failure or starvation.

Laceration: Rip/tear in the skin or another tissue (e.g. a tendon).

Laminitis: See "Founder".

Membrane: An outer covering

Mucus Membrane: Fluid secreting linings of the mouth, nose, throat, reproductive tracts.

Myelitis: Spinal cord inflammation.

Narcolepsy: Disorder of the brain which causes animal to appear to fall asleep inappropriately (e.g. while eating). A form of epilepsy.

Neoplasm: Abnormal growth, tumor.

Ophthalmic/Ophthalmologic: Pertaining to the eye.

Patent Urachus: Open connection between the urinary bladder and the umbilical cord in a newborn foal.

Pleuritis: Inflammation of the tissues lining the chest and covering the lungs (usually caused by infection).

Renal: Pertaining to the kidney.

Rhino/Rhinopneumonitis: A common respiratory viral infection in horses.

Salmonella: A common bacterial infection of the intestinal tract.

Sclera: The "white" of the eye.

Subcutaneous: Under the skin.

Tetanus: A rigid paralysis caused by toxins produced when a wound is infected with the organism Clostridium tetani.

Toxoid: A "tamed" version of a toxin that is injected into the animal to stimulate his immune system to produce antibodies that will be ready to guard against that specific poison.

Toxin: A poisonous substance, harmful substance.

Tracheotomy: Making a hole in the trachea ("windpipe").

Tracheostomy: Inserting something into the trachea to keep a surgical opening open.

Ulcer: Any defect in the surface of a tissue, usually caused by surface tissues being injured and defective in some way.

INDEX